The Dose–Response Relation
in Pharmacology

*The year 1979 marks the hundredth anniversary of Albert Einstein's birth. It seems fitting that this work, appearing this year, should acknowledge the achievements of this distinguished scientist and humanitarian who so elevated the public's opinions of science and scientists.*

Ronald J. Tallarida          Leonard S. Jacob

# The Dose–Response Relation in Pharmacology

# in Pharmacology

*With 108 illustrations*

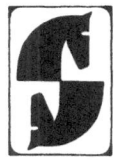

Springer-Verlag    New York    Heidelberg    Berlin

**Ronald J. Tallarida, Ph.D.**
Professor of Pharmacology
Temple University School of Medicine
Philadelphia, Pennsylvania 19140

**Leonard S. Jacob, M.D., Ph.D.**
Faculty, Departments of Anesthesiology and Pharmacology
University of Pennsylvania School of Medicine
Philadelphia, Pennsylvania 19104
and
Visiting Assistant Professor of Pharmacology
Medical College of Pennsylvania
Philadelphia, Pennsylvania 19129

**Library of Congress Cataloging in Publication Data**

Tallarida, Ronald J.

    Dose–response relation in pharmacology.

    Includes index.
    1.  Drugs—Dose–response relationship.    2.  Drug
receptors.  I.  Jacob, Leonard S., joint author.
II.  Title.  [DNLM:  1.  Dose–response relationship,
Drug.  QV38.3 T147d]
RM301.8.T34        615'.7        79-13824

ISBN-13: 978-1-4684-6267-8      e-ISBN-13: 978-1-4684-6265-4
DOI: 10.1007/978-1-4684-6265-4

## To Alexander Gero

*who introduced us to drug–receptor theory*
*and to each other*

# Preface

This book is designed to meet the modern need for a better understanding of drug–receptor interaction as applied to the gathering and interpretation of dose–response data. It is an introduction suitable for any student who has had a first course in pharmacology. This book is an extension of the pharmacology course into one area of what is now known as molecular pharmacology. The material included is an outgrowth of courses that we have given in recent years to health-science students in several professional schools and universities.

The area of drug–receptor theory, although just a part of molecular pharmacology, is already very broad. One major line of investigation is concerned with the chemical and structural nature of specific receptors and with efforts to isolate specific receptors. Another line of investigation is concerned with the kinetic theories of drug–receptor interaction, the effort there being to provide a general theory that is applicable to wide classes of drugs. We have chosen to deal with the latter.

There are several reasons for our choice of topics. First, the information is very practical; that is, it permits one to use properly and consistently terms such as "efficacy," "partial agonist," "pure antagonist," "potency," "$pA_2$," etc., when describing drug action. Second, many students fail to appreciate the differences in and the limitations of the various theories, beginning with the classical theory of A. J. Clark, on up to the very recent allosteric theories. Such differences are important, of course, in the consistent interpretation of experimental results. (For example, to classify a drug as a "strong agonist" and to proceed to find its dissociation constant from a Lineweaver–Burk plot is inconsistent.) Third, knowledge of these theories is a prerequisite for understanding much current research, including efforts aimed at chemical and structural identification of receptors. Finally, most textbooks of pharmacology, necessarily thick with drug facts, can devote little attention to this subject; hence, it is not easy to find these topics under one cover in a form that is suitable for the beginner.

It is impossible here to sketch, even briefly, or even to cite, the tremendous development in our field. We make no claim, therefore, at completeness in our discussions. We have chosen, instead, to use information from the literature in order to illustrate the methods, experimental and theoretical, needed to understand the principles. The emphasis throughout is on principles. Nevertheless, we chose our sources carefully. Thus, the references can both serve as sources of greater detail and introduce the reader to a specialized area of interest.

The first five chapters deal with definitions and theories. The objective in these chapters is methodology for the collection and presentation of dose–response data, and the interpretation of these data. To this end we have included the most important theories of drug action.

Much of the material in Chapter 2 and the discussions of calculus in Appendix C represent a review of some rather basic mathematical concepts. The topics presented are those that are needed in the several theories that form the basis for interpreting dose–response data. We have included this material in order to make the book reasonably self-contained. No attempt was made to give a mathematically rigorous treatment, since most readers of this book will have had formal courses in mathematics at this level. We applied the same reasoning in our selection and treatment of the statistical topics in Chapter 4.

Chapter 6 is in many ways a separate division of the book; in a sense, it may be considered "Part II." The chapter contains dose–response curves for a number of pharmacological preparations that are used widely in student and professional laboratories. The drugs discussed may be thought of as prototypes against which other drugs may be compared. This material should provide the reader with basic information sufficient to start one in the use of a new preparation, either for original research or for teaching purposes.

Appendixes A–C contain numerical tables, the compositions of various solutions, molecular weights of selected drugs, and a brief review of calculus.

This book is not meant to be an exhaustive treatise on current theories, nor is it strictly a textbook. Although combining features of each, it is, we hope, a book for students and professionals that may narrow the gap that separates experimentalists and theoreticians in one part of this multidisciplined subject.

We would like to thank Miss Ellen Geller, Dr. Anthony Mucci, and Dr. Rodney Murray for their help with the proofreading, and also our fine typists, Dolores McMonigle, Theresa Valera, and Susan Wendling. We wish to express our appreciation to Drs. Martin Adler, Concetta Harakal, and Malcolm MacNab, who provided us with some of the data, and to all the investigators whose works we have borrowed from. Also, we are grateful for the very generous assistance we received from our friends in the Pharmacology Department at Temple Medical School who helped in so many ways in the preparation of this work, especially Dr. Alan Cowan, Robert Kent, Paul McGonigle, Frank Porreca, Robert Raffa, Mary Jane Robinson, and Mark Watson.

Finally, we would like to thank Dr. Alexander Gero, to whom we have dedicated this book. Not only have we learned much from Dr. Gero, but also his excitement about the subject continues to be a constant source of inspiration to us.

Ronald J. Tallarida
Leonard S. Jacob

# Contents

# The Dose–Response Relation

## Chapter 1

*I often say that when you can measure what you are speaking
about, and express it in numbers, you know something about it; but
when you cannot express it in numbers, your knowledge is of a
meagre and unsatisfactory kind; it may be the beginning of
knowledge, but you have scarcely, in your thoughts, advanced to
that stage of Science, whatever the matter may be.*

LORD KELVIN (1824–1907)

## Introduction

Molecular pharmacology is concerned with studies of basic mechanisms of
drug actions on biological systems. It considers molecules as the basic functional
units both of the drug and of the system on which the drug acts. Its objective
is to determine and interpret the relation between biological activity and the
structure of molecules or groups of molecules. Not only is it the level of investigation that defines this modern topic in pharmacology, but also it is the emphasis
on precise *measurement* in experimental studies.

In this book we will be concerned with the gathering and use of measures
of drug dose and response, with the presentation of these measured values
in various ways, and with the interpretation of the measurements using the
several drug–receptor theories. The scope of the book is limited to concepts
that are applicable to drugs in general, and not to specific drug–effector systems.
There is much more to molecular pharmacology and to drug–receptor theory
than we can present. We have not included such topics as structure–activity
relationships, or the mapping of specific receptors. We refer the reader to the
literature on these exciting topics. The material we have included is, we hope,
very practical because of its wide applicability, intellectually satisfying and,
therefore, important in the training of the modern pharmacologist, whatever
his or her role might be.

## The Dose–Response Relation

It is known that even primitive man associated specific drugs with specific disease states. Implicit in this association was the question of how much drug is needed in order to achieve the desired effect. *This correspondence between the amount of drug and the magnitude of the effect produced is an example of a dose–effect or dose–response relation.* In modern pharmacology, this relation is important, both for therapeutic purposes and as a first step in understanding mechanism. The determination of the dose–response relation for a particular drug–effector combination, and the interpretation of this relation within the framework of different theories of drug action are the main objectives of this monograph.

In practice, one studies drug effects in the intact organism or in any component of the organism such as an organ, a cell, or a cellular component. The effect is always some measurable change in the component under study. The effect may be the immediate molecular event, it may be a secondary event, or it may be the composite of several events, an effect which is far removed from the molecular level. Unfortunately we do not know in many cases what these intimate molecular events are, or how they relate to each other or to the observable effect being studied. Thus modern pharmacologists study drug effects at several levels: molecular, cellular, organ, organ system, and organism. For example, a drug that contracts skeletal muscle causes a release of calcium ions from their storage sites (a rather intimate effect); the $Ca^{2+}$ combines with troponin, permitting the formation of cross bridges between actin and myosin which produce contraction. If the muscle in question is one that is involved in breathing, then the respiration of the organism will be affected. Any one of these effects, $Ca^{2+}$ flux, muscle tension, augmentation of respiration, or any other event in the process may be taken as the drug effect.

As another example, suppose the drug effect being studied is the change in pupil size. This effect depends on the more elementary effects, such as the degree of contracture of the opposing muscles, radial dilator and circular constricting, which determine pupil aperture. This is a good example of an effect that is the result of two effects, neither of which is very intimate.

Although one can study an effect produced by a drug and determine a dose–response relation, great care must be exercised in connecting this relation with the mechanism at the molecular level. Indeed, much of the controversy that surrounds the several current theories of drug action results from unfounded assumptions connecting effects with bound drug. These theories are discussed in Chapter 3.

Regardless of the level of study, a drug effect should have two properties. First, it should be measurable. Second, it should have the value zero when the dose is zero. Thus a plot of effect versus dose should result in a curve that passes through the origin of the coordinate system. The dose, or concentration, being the *independent variable*, is usually plotted on the abscissa. The effect is then

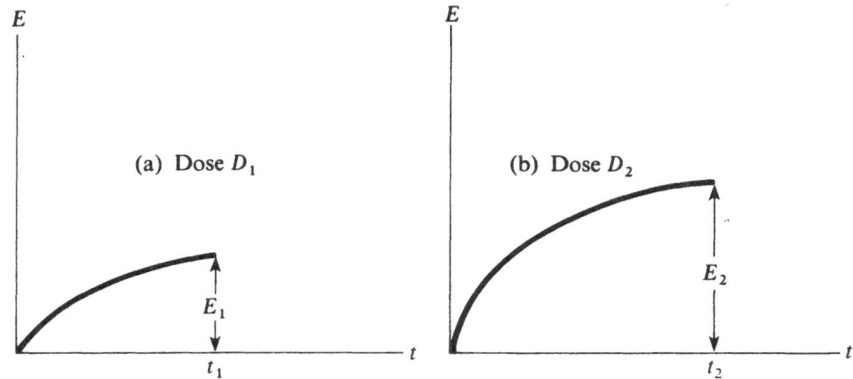

**Figure 1.1** Response as a function of time and dose. $E_1$ and $E_2$ are equilibrium responses.

the *dependent variable* and is plotted on the ordinate. As the observed effect is usually not instantaneous, but takes some time to appear after administration of the drug, the effect is properly stated to depend on both the time and the dose; hence, the effect will be a function of time and dose: $E = f(t, D)$.

We often take the peak effect, or the equilibrium effect produced by a given dose, without concern for the time course of development of the effect. This practice yields a *time-independent* dose–response relation.

Figure 1.1a is a plot of response $E$ versus time after a dose $D_1$ administered at time $t = 0$. The effect increases in time, reaching an equilibrium value $E_1$ at time $t_1$. If one gives a larger dose $D_2$, the effect reaches a larger equilibrium value $E_2$ at some time $t_2$, as in Figure 1.1b. Thus the response is *graded*. In general, for increasing doses, $D_1, D_2, \ldots, D_i$, we observe increasing effects, $E_1, E_2, \ldots, E_i$. Eventually a dose $D_n$ is reached beyond which no further increase in effect occurs; we denote by $E_{max}$ this maximum possible effect. The totality of pairs $(D_1, E_1), (D_2, E_2), \ldots, (D_i, E_i), \ldots, (D_n, E_{max})$, gives a graded dose–response curve for this drug–effector combination as in Figure 1.2. It should be noted that, although there is a natural upper bound for the effect, there is no corresponding upper limit for the dose. We have denoted by $D_n$ that dose above which no detectable increase in effect is achieved with this particular drug, but the curve continues, remaining flat, for dose ranges above $D_n$.

A point of the curve that has particular significance in the theory to follow is that which corresponds to a half-maximal or 50% response. *The dose which gives* $E = \frac{1}{2}E_{max}$ *is called* $D_{50}$. In actual experiments the value of $D_{50}$ is determined from the smooth curve that connects the data points. (Occasionally $D_{50}$ happens to be one of the administered doses.) The height of the plateau of the curve equals $E_{max}$ and is taken to be a measure of the *efficacy* of the drug. The left-to-right position of the dose–response curve, indicating the magnitude of the effect for a given dose, is a measure of the drug's *potency*. Thus two drugs which are qualitatively the same in producing a particular effect may differ in

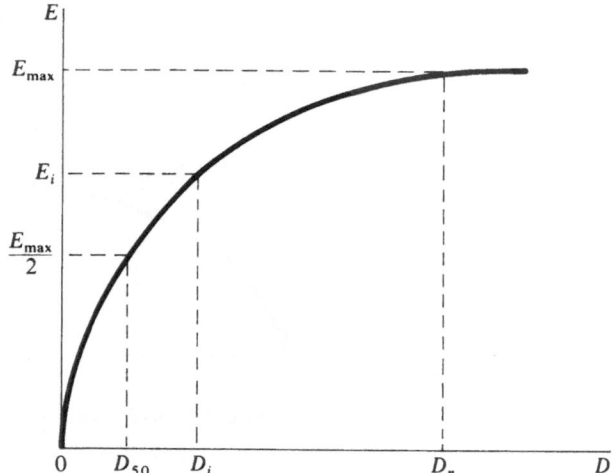

**Figure 1.2** The graded dose–response curve. Each value, such as $E_i$, is the equilibrium effect for dose $D_i$. The dose that produces a half-maximal effect is denoted "$D_{50}$."

either efficacy or potency, or both. Figure 1.3 illustrates the concepts of efficacy and potency for two drugs, A and B, that produce qualitatively identical effects.

Efficacy is a measure of the intrinsic ability of a drug to produce an effect and is, therefore, useful for therapeutic purposes; potency is generally considered less important therapeutically since it usually makes little difference whether one has to take 1 mg or 10 mg in order to achieve a certain level of effect. Potency is influenced by many factors such as absorption, metabolism, etc. On the other hand, efficacy is related to a more fundamental action of the drug.

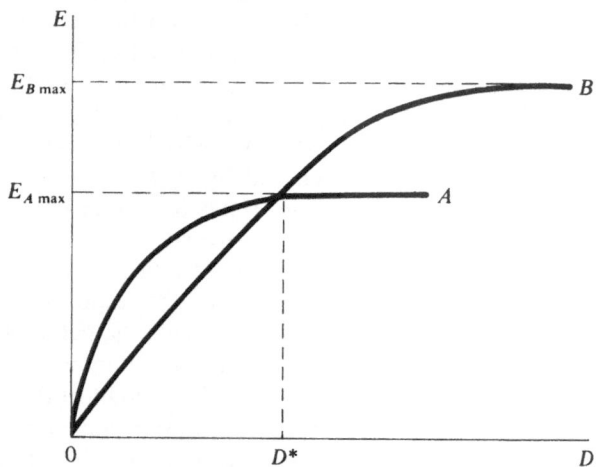

**Figure 1.3** Efficacy and potency. Drug B has the greater efficacy. Over the range of doses 0–$D^*$, drug A has the greater potency.

## Methods of Plotting Dose–Response Curves

In this section we illustrate some commonly used methods in plotting graded dose–response data. Several examples follow.

Figure 1.4 illustrates a dose–response relation in which analgesia in the rat (measured as ability to withstand tail compression) is related to the dose of morphine administered. Two facts of the plotting are noteworthy. The first is that the response is expressed as a *percent of the maximum response*. Second, the calibration of the dose-axis (the abscissa) is *linear*, that is, equal intervals on the scale correspond to the same dose increment. In Figure 1.5, we have another dose–response curve for morphine in the rat; in this case, the response is the increase in convulsive-seizure threshold (i.e., the time, in seconds, before the animal convulses after receiving a convulsive stimulant). Here again, both the ordinate and the abscissa have linear scales; however, the response is presented in *absolute units* rather than as a percent of the maximum. Of course, one could convert the ordinate to percent of $E_{max}$ by dividing each $E$ by $E_{max}$ and multiplying by 100. The process is called *normalization* and is a common method in the presentation of dose–response data.

In Figure 1.6, we have illustrated the dose–response curve derived from data obtained in an isolated muscle strip of rabbit thoracic aorta contracted

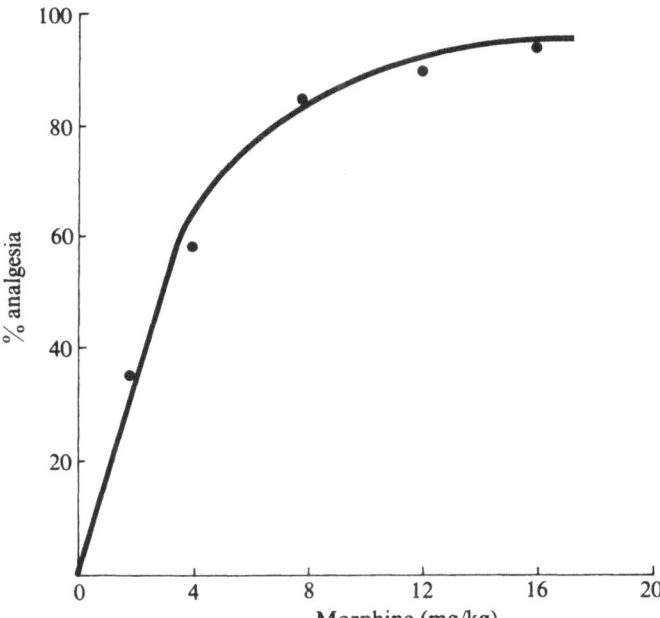

**Figure 1.4** The analgesic effect of subcutaneous injections of morphine in the rat. From Harakal et al.[7]

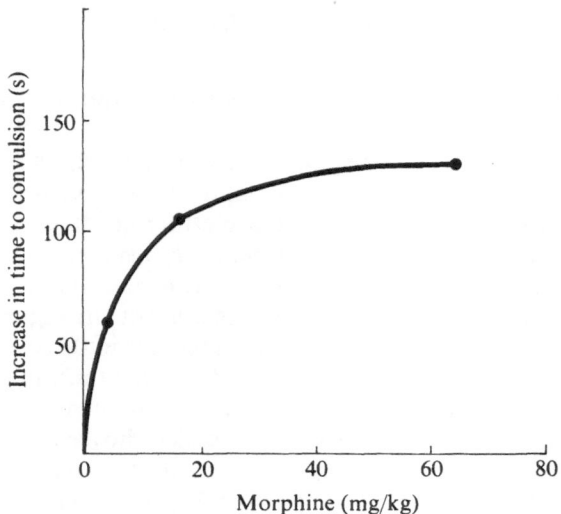

**Figure 1.5** The effect of morphine on seizure threshold in the rat. From Adler et al.[1]

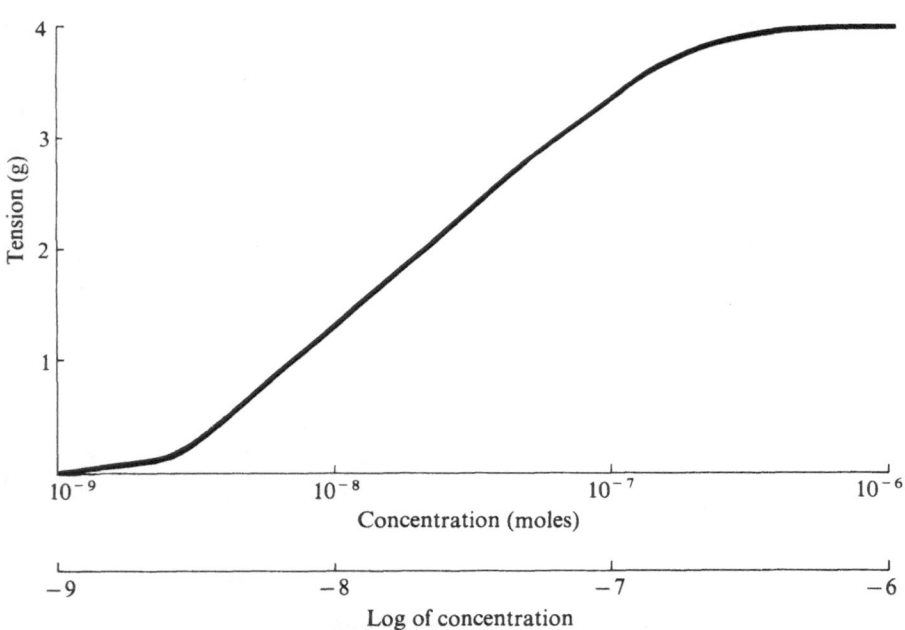

**Figure 1.6** Dose–response curve for norepinephrine on isolated thoracic aorta of the rabbit, illustrating the use of a logarithmic scale for the dose. From Tallarida et al.[12]

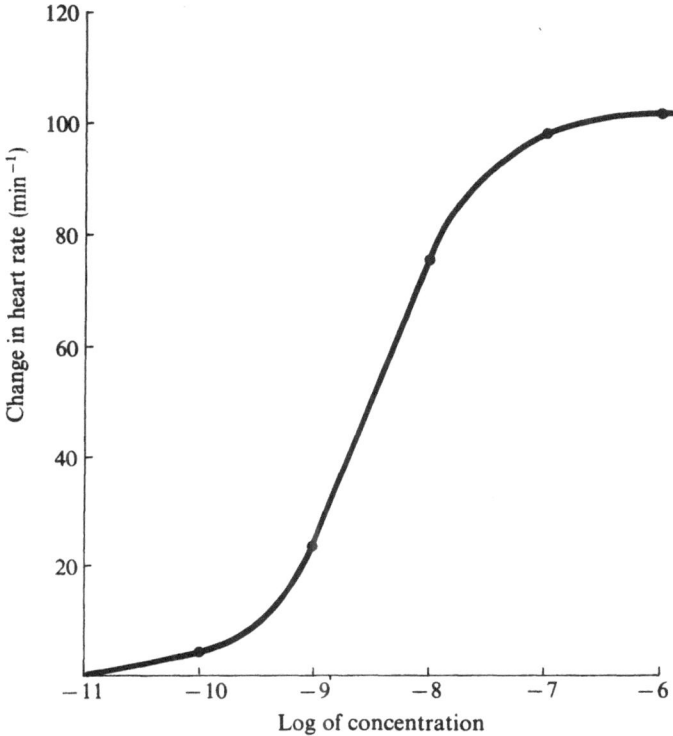

**Figure 1.7** A drug-induced effect is some measurable change in the system. In this case the effect is the *change* in heart rate produced by isoproterenol. A logarithmic scale is used for the dose.

with norepinephrine. The response is developed tension, in g,* under conditions of constant length (isometric tension). On the abscissa is the concentration of norepinephrine in molar units. A noteworthy feature of this plot is that the horizontal scale is not calibrated linearly, that is, equal divisions do not represent equal increments in the drug concentration. This representation is often used when the range of doses is large, in this case, $10^{-9}$–$10^{-6}$ $M$.

It is seen that the abscissa in Figure 1.6 is calibrated *logarithmically*, that is, the same concentration scale could be expressed as log(concentration) with the numbers, $-9$, $-8$, $-7$, $-6$, used as labels, as shown in the figure.† Because

---

* What is measured is the developed *force*. The gram is a unit of *mass*, not force. The unit of force is the *dyne* or the *newton*; the practice of expressing force in units of gram is common in pharmacology. To convert grams to dynes we multiply grams by 980, the gravitational acceleration, and 1 newton $= 10^5$ dynes.

† The negative common logarithm of the $D_{50}$ concentration is often used. It has been termed "$pD_2$."

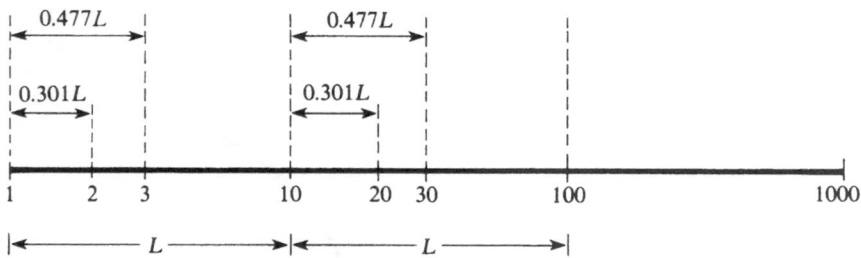

**Figure 1.8** The construction of a logarithmic scale.

this method is so common, we shall discuss the construction of logarithmic scales at the end of this section.

Figure 1.7 shows the change in the heart rate of a dog as a function of increasing doses of isoproterenol. Note that the effect is the *change* in rate, $\Delta$ H. R., not the rate itself. The control rate (i.e., the rate with no drug) was 85/min. The concentration range was $1 \times 10^{-11}$ $M$ to $3.2 \times 10^{-6}$, producing a maximum effect $\Delta$ H. R. = 102/min.

The dose–response relation can often be approximated by a function of the type

$$E = \frac{C_1 D}{C_2 + D},$$
(1.1)

where $C_1$ and $C_2$ are numerical constants that have a particular significance in so-called classical theory of drug action (see Chap. 3). If the pairs $(D, E)$ are plotted in rectangular coordinates with *linear* scales, the plotted points yield a *hyperbolic* curve. [The equation $E = C_1 D/(C_2 + D)$ graphs as a hyperbola.] If the abscissa has a logarithmic scale the curve takes on a *sigmoid* or *S*-shape.

A logarithmic scale is constructed as in Figure 1.8. The major subdivision has some length $L$, representing a *decade* or *cycle*. Note that this same length $L$ divides the intervals 1 to 10, 10 to 100, 100 to 1000, etc. Intermediate points are marked as follows: for example, to mark "2" in the first cycle, or "20" in the second cycle, one multiplies $L$ by log 2 or $L \times 0.301$. The number 3 (or 30) is located from log 3 $\times$ $L$ or $0.477L$, and each integer up to 9, is located in the same manner.

## Drug Antagonism

It is generally held that most drugs act by combining with some specific cell component in order to produce an effect. This component of the cell has been referred to as a *receptor*; the idea is similar to that of enzyme–substrate interaction in which the enzyme and the substrate react to form an enzyme–substrate

(a) Physiological antagonism

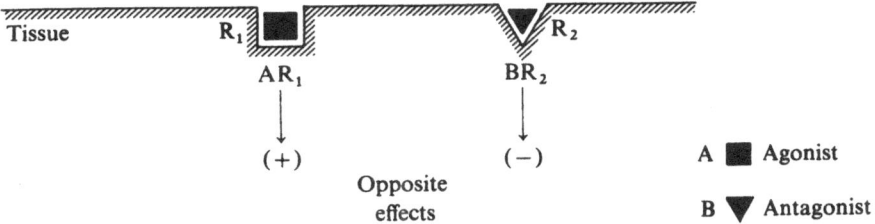

(b) Pharmacological antagonism

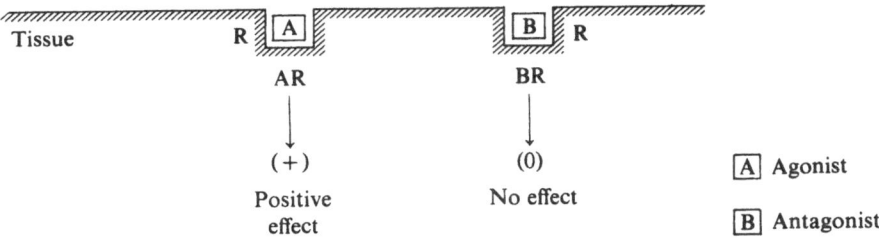

**Figure 1.9** Schematic diagram of antagonisms. (a) Physiological antagonism—two receptors, opposite effects; (b) pharmacological antagonism—a single receptor, but drug B lacks "intrinsic activity."

complex. In the case of a drug and its receptor, a drug–receptor complex is formed, and this complex somehow provides the stimulus for the resulting effect. Such an active drug is said to have *intrinsic activity* and is termed an *agonist*. It is well known that some drugs act in association with an agonist in such a way that the effect of the agonist is reduced or even abolished. Such agents are called *antagonists*. Drug antagonisms may result from different mechanisms but may be broadly classified according to whether the antagonist combines with the same receptor as that of the agonist or with a different receptor. The former case in which both the agonist and the antagonist combine with the same receptor is called *pharmacological antagonism*; when the receptors are different the antagonism is called *physiological* or *functional* (see Fig. 1.9).

A pharmacological antagonist, though having affinity for the receptor, may have no ability to initiate activity of its own, that is, it may have no *intrinsic activity*, or its intrinsic activity may be small compared to that of the agonist. Thus, the presence of the antagonist reduces the magnitude of the effect of the agonist. In some cases, this inhibition may be overcome completely by increasing the concentration of the agonist. Such is the case, for example, with isoproterenol

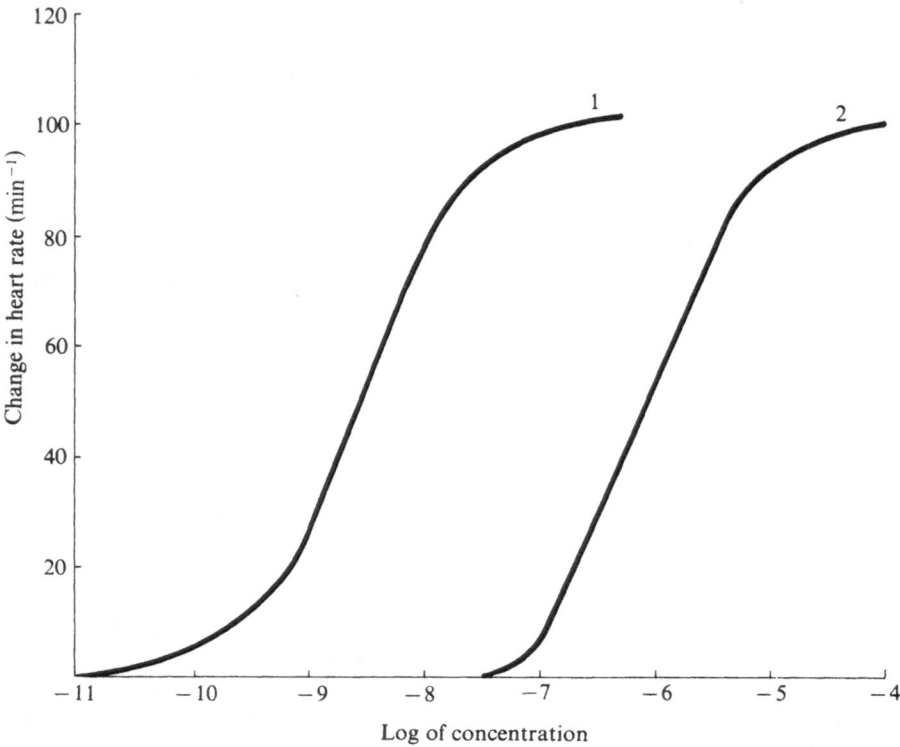

**Figure 1.10** Competitive antagonism of isoproterenol by propranolol. Both curves represent the effects of increasing doses of the agonist, isoproterenol. Curve 2 results from pretreatment with propranolol. With logarithmic dose scales, competitive antagonists give rise to parallel curves having the same maximum. From Blinks.[4]

and propranolol as shown in Figure 1.10 in which the effect is the increase in heart rate. Curve 1 is the log dose–response curve for isoproterenol alone, and curve 2 is the result of propranolol plus isoproterenol, producing a shift in the curve. Note that *the antagonism is completely overcome by increasing the concentration of isoproterenol* and that the curves are *parallel*. Following the analogy with enzyme–substrate reactions, we call this type of antagonism *surmountable* or *competitive*. Thus, propranolol is a competitive antagonist of isoproterenol. Many examples of competitive antagonism exist—atropine and "muscarinic" acetylcholine receptors, naloxone and morphine receptors, and phentolamine and α-adrenergic receptors (Fig. 1.11). Competitive antagonists have several important properties of which the following two are important in the present discussion: (1) They give rise to *parallel* log dose–response curves, and (2) the antagonism is surmountable so that the curves attain the *same maximum effect*.

In contrast to competitive antagonists whose inhibitory action is *reversible*,

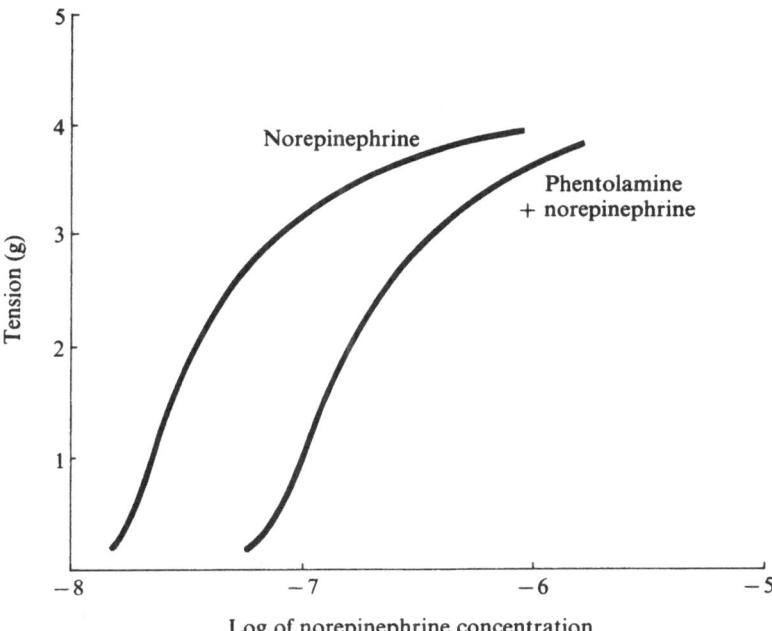

**Figure 1.11** Competitive antagonism of norepinephrine by phentolamine on isolated rabbit thoracic aorta. From Jacob.[8]

some pharmacological antagonists either have very high affinity for the receptor or produce irreversible chemical changes in the receptor. In either case *further addition of the agonist does not restore the full effect*. This kind of antagonism is called *noncompetitive*. Such inhibition may be partial, blocking only a fraction of the receptors, or it may be complete. An example of noncompetitive antagonism is that which occurs between norepinephrine and phenoxybenzamine. This is illustrated in Figure 1.12 in which we have plotted complete dose-response curves for isometric tension in vascular smooth muscle as a function of the norepinephrine concentration, in the absence of phenoxybenzamine, and in the presence of several fixed concentrations of phenoxybenzamine. At any one of the antagonist concentrations, the full norepinephrine effect is not achieved, and at sufficiently high concentrations of phenoxybenzamine, the norepinephrine effect is completely abolished.

In physiological or functional antagonism the drugs antagonize each other by acting on different receptors that produce opposite effects. For example, histamine produces a contraction and epinephrine a relaxation on bronchial muscle. Another example is the antagonism between the sympathetic neurotransmitter, norepinephrine, and the parasympathetic neurotransmitter, acetylcholine, on pupil size. In the latter case, not only are the receptors different,

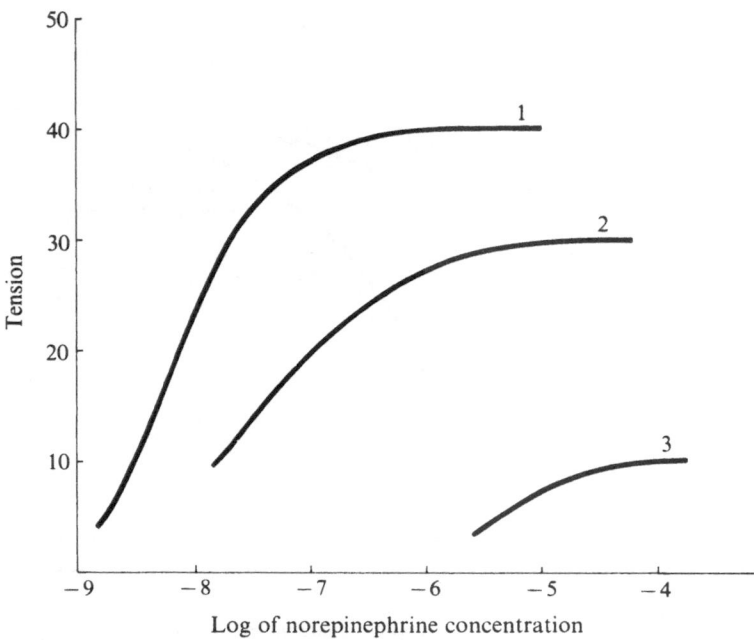

**Figure 1.12** Noncompetitive antagonism of norepinephrine by two different doses of phenoxybenzamine on rabbit thoracic aorta. The effect is developed tension in millinewtons. Curve 2 results from $5 \times 10^{-9}M$ phenoxybenzamine, and curve 3 from $5 \times 10^{-8}M$ antagonist. In each case the full agonist effect cannot be produced.

but also the muscles are different. In each muscle the effect is contraction, but the anatomical arrangement is such that one muscle (the sphincter pupillae) constricts, whereas the other (the radial dilator) dilates. In most cases of physiological antagonism, the dose–response curves will more nearly resemble those of noncompetitive antagonism. It should be kept in mind, however, that when the nature of the antagonism of one drug by the other is unknown, the dose–response curves alone are not sufficient to make a conclusion as to whether the agents are acting on the same or on different receptors. Parallel log dose–response curves, however, would strongly suggest (but not prove) competitive antagonism. If the curves are not parallel, there may be either two different receptors or a single receptor that has been irreversibly altered (noncompetitive). These points will be amplified in Chapter 3 in which we discuss the kinetics of drug–receptor interactions.

Regardless of the competitive or noncompetitive nature of the antagonism, and regardless of the mechanism, it is frequently desirable to determine doses (or concentrations) of the agonist that produce equal effects. Figure 1.13 illustrates a situation in which a level of effect, $E_1$, is produced by agonist concentration $D_1$ when agonist alone is used, but a greater agonist concentra-

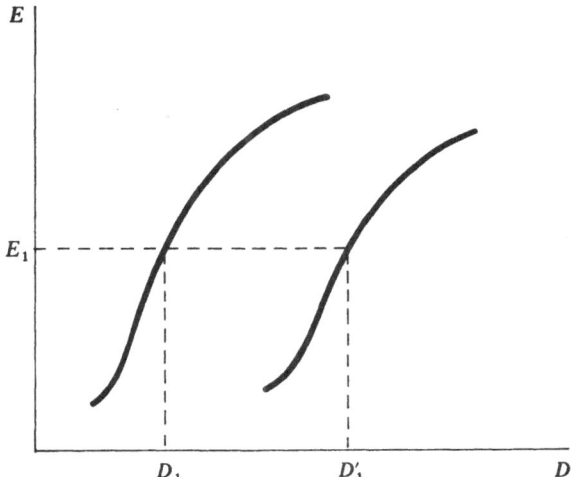

**Figure 1.13** In the presence of the antagonist, a larger dose $D_1'$ of agonist is required to produce the same effect.

tion, $D_1'$, is required when in the presence of the antagonist. The term *dose ratio* is often used for the ratio $D_1'/D_1$. This ratio may be constant throughout the range of effects, or it may vary. The significance of the constancy or variability of this ratio will be discussed in Chapter 3.

Evidence for the existence of specific receptors in a tissue comes from several lines of investigation. For example, it has been found in numerous studies that many drugs can be antagonized selectively, meaning that one agent may block the effect (say, contraction of muscle) of one agonist, but not have any effect on the action of other agonists producing the same effect. It is no accident, therefore, that our first use of the term "receptor" occurs in this section in which we discuss drug antagonism. There are other characteristics of the action of drugs that support the receptor concept,[13] namely (1) they act at low concentrations, (2) their activity is easily influenced by changes in their chemical structure, and (3) the inhibitory action of the antagonists is also influenced by changes in the chemical structure. When a drug action is mediated through a specific receptor we call the drug action *specific*, in contrast to nonspecific drug action (such as the actions of the volatile anesthetics). Even though we do not know the physicochemical nature of most receptors, some are "known" to us by a rather elaborate classification scheme.

A good example of such a classification is that used for adrenoreceptors. These are classified according to their ligand specificity, the most important classification being $\alpha$ and $\beta$. Ahlquist[2,3] classified these in terms of the order of potency of a series of adrenergic agonists in eliciting certain responses. For the $\alpha$-receptor the order relation is in terms of potency: norepinephrine > epinephrine > phenylephrine > isoproterenol. For the $\beta$-receptor the order is isoproterenol > epinephrine > norepinephrine > phenylephrine. Furchgott[6] sharpened this classification by including the susceptibility to specific blockers such as propranolol for $\beta$ actions and phentolamine for $\alpha$ actions. These types of classification are based on pharmacological experimentation. Other classifications are based on biochemical events coupled to these receptors as discussed in the review by Levitzki.[10] The use of both pharmacological and biochemical criteria for classifying receptors is discussed in the review (on dopamine receptors) by Kebabian and Calne.[9]

Some of the older evidence for the existence of specific receptors is discussed in Chapter 3. A relatively new line of investigation in the classification of receptors uses radiolabeled agents. This topic is discussed Chapter 5.

## Use of Dose–Response Curves

Dose–response relations are useful in many ways. They provide valuable information regarding the efficacy and potency in producing a given effect. It is a fact, however, that most drugs produce not just one, but a myriad of effects. Thus, one can determine a dose–response relation for each one of the several effects produced by a given drug. These various dose–effect relations are frequently different, producing curves with different shapes and, hence, different values of $D_{50}$, potency, etc. One should be cautious, therefore, in formulating theories of drug–receptor interaction based on dose–effect curves alone. Usually one needs to have a good deal of other information about the action of a drug before it is possible to make conclusions about mechanism. Generally speaking, the more complicated the effect, the more difficult it is to relate dose–effect data to drug–receptor mechanisms. That is, if a drug effect is rather intimate, such as a change in ionic conductance in a muscle membrane, an effect that precedes muscle contraction, it is safer to draw conclusions regarding mechanism that it is for a more distal effect, or for an effect that is a composite of several effects. We may, therefore, distinguish between *drug-dependent* and *drug-independent* effects as illustrated in Figure 1.14. When, however, information about the drug mechanism is known, it is possible to use dose–effect information, and certain theoretical assumptions, to draw quantitative and qualitative conclusions about drug–receptor interactions.

Although theories of drug action are not built on the shape of dose–response curves alone, there are situations in which it is useful to describe such curves mathematically. Such situations arise when one wishes to compare potency ratios or efficacies among several agonists or when the effects of antagonists are being studied (p. 61). Various forms of the *logistic equation* have been used in this kind of analysis.[5,14] One form of the logistic equation is given by

$$Y = \frac{-a}{1 + (x/c)^b} + a. \tag{1.2}$$

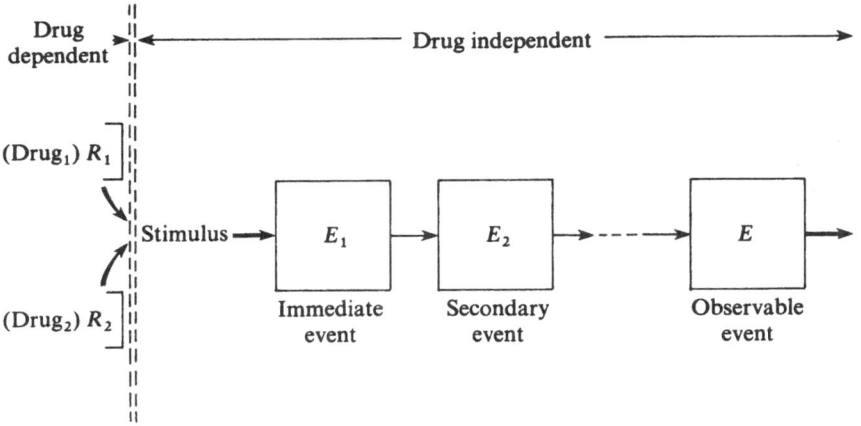

**Figure 1.14** The relation between the stimulus and response is a property of the system and is independent of the drug. Drugs differ in their ability to produce stimuli.

This equation, often used for bioassay, yields a sigmoidal (S-shaped) curve when plotted on a logarithmic abscissa. When applied to dose–response data, $Y$ is the response, $x$ is the concentration, $a$ is the response at saturation, $c$ is the concentration that produces a half-maximal response, and $b$ is a constant related to the slope (see also p. 8).

## Enhancement of Drug Action

In contrast to antagonism of one drug by the other, there are numerous situations in which the presence of a second drug causes an increase in the effect produced. For example, norepinephrine constricts most arteries; the peptide, angiotensin II, also constricts arteries. If the two are present together, the contribution of each produces a *summation* of effects.

In some situations the enhancement of effect produced by a second drug acting with the first may be more than simple algebraic summation. This kind of interaction is referred to as *potentiation* or *synergism*. A frequently used example of synergism is the diuretic action of the combination ammonium chloride and mercurial ion. In this case the mechanism of the potentiation is clear. Both are diuretics but, in addition, ammonium chloride acidifies the urine, resulting in a situation which promotes the ionization of the mercurial. There are many other examples of potentiation in which the mechanism is known, a common mechanism being that in which the second drug promotes release of a substance that is similar in action to that of the first drug.

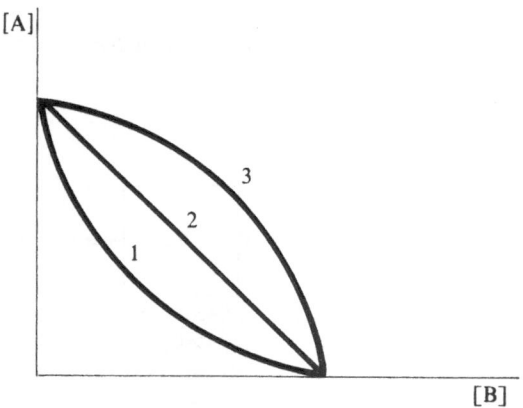

**Figure 1.15** Isoboes—curve 2 has slope −1.

At the level of specific receptors a possible model for potentiation of effects pictures the presence of drug 1 as having the effect of *sensitizing* the receptor for drug 2. Thus we have two receptors with two drugs, and one of the receptors is capable of initiating more than its usual stimulus, the effects being now more than the algebraic sum.

Regardless of which mechanism of enhancement is in operation, a graphical method first introduced by Loewe and Muischnek[11] is sometimes used to display the interaction. This method used loci of identical effects of a combination of two drugs. A constant level of effect is selected, say 50 % of $E_{max}$. The sets of concentrations of drugs A and B which, as a mixture, produce this effect are plotted, [A] against [B], producing a curve called an *isobole*. Strict additivity, which means [A] + [B] = a constant, results in a curve of slope −1 as seen in Figure 1.15 (curve 2). If, however, the mixture requires greater concentrations than expected by simple additivity in order to achieve this effect, then the isobole is concave downward as in curve 3, meaning some antagonism is present. If the concentrations in the mixture turn out to be lower than those for additivity, there is an enhancement of action that has been called *potentiation* or *synergism*. In this case the isobole will be concave upward as in curve 1.

## References

1. Adler, M. W., Lin, C. H., Keinath, S. H., Braverman, S., and Geller, E. B.: J. Pharmacol. Exp. Ther., *198*:655, 1976.
2. Ahlquist, R. P.: Am. J. Physiol., *153*:586, 1948.
3. Ahlquist, R. P.: Ann. N.Y. Acad. Sci., *139*:549, 1967.
4. Blinks, J. R.: Ann. N.Y. Acad. Sci., *139*:673, 1967.
5. De Lean, A., Munson, P. J., and Rodbard, D.: Am. J. Physiol., *235*:E97, 1978.
6. Furchgott, R. F.: In *Handbook of Experimental Pharmacology. 33* (H. Blascho, and E. Muscholl, eds.) New York, Springer-Verlag, 1972, pp. 283–335.

7. Harakal, C., Tallarida, R. J., Geller, E. B., Biunno, I., and Adler, M. W.: The Pharmacologist, *18*:174, 1976.
8. Jacob, L. S.: Ph.D. thesis, Temple University, Philadelphia, Pa., 1974.
9. Kebabian, J. W., and Calne, D. B.: Nature, *277*:93, 1979.
10. Levitzki, A.: Rev. Physiol. Biochem. Pharmacol., *82*:1, 1978.
11. Loewe, S., and Muischnek, H.: Arch. Exp. Pathol. Pharmakol., *114*:313, 1926.
12. Tallarida, R. J., Sevy, R. W., Harakal, C., and Loughnane, M.H.: *IEEE* Trans. Biomed. Engineering, *22*:493, 1975.
13. Waud, D. R.: Pharmacol. Rev. *20*:49, 1968.
14. Waud, D. R., and Parker, R. B.: J. Pharmacol. Exp. Ther., *117*:13, 1970.

# Functions and Relations

## Chapter 2

## Mathematical Symbols and Conventions

The mathematical symbols used in this book are in common usage in the literature dealing with the quantitative aspects of pharmacology and, for the most part, conform to standard mathematical usage. In our choice of variables, however, we preferred, in some instances, to use single letter symbols such as $x$, $y$, and $E$ as variables, rather than the more descriptive symbols such as "conc." (for concentration), "vol" (for volume), "Eff" (for effect), etc. Our usage was dictated by a desire to reduce the bulk of notation in situations in which there was some reasonable amount of manipulation.

Mathematical symbols which, though standard, are worthy of a reminder, are discussed below along with certain basic mathematical concepts.

The symbols $\doteqdot$ and $\approx$ are each used to mean "approximately equal." Thus, $\pi \approx 3.14$, and $\sqrt{2} \approx 1.414$, or $\sqrt{2} \doteqdot 1.414$. The symbol $>$ means "greater than," and $<$ means "less than," whereas $\geq$ means "greater than or equal to" and $\leq$ means "less than or equal to." The radical $\sqrt{(\ \ )}$ always means the *positive* square root of the *nonnegative* number inside the parentheses. For example, $\sqrt{(16)} = 4$, *never* $(-4)$. The symbol $\sum_{i=1}^{n} (\ \ )$ is used for repetitive addition. The letter $i$ is the index of summation and increases by 1 as we go from term to term.

The starting value (1) and the finishing value ($n$) for the index are part of the notation. Thus $\sum_{i=1}^{10} a_i$ means $a_1 + a_2 + \cdots + a_{10}$. If the variable associated with $\sum$ is *not* subscripted, then that variable is added the number of times indicated by the index. For example, $\sum_{i=1}^{5} b = b + b + b + b + b = 5b$.

The symbol $|a|$ stands for the *absolute value* or magnitude of the number $a$. Thus $|a|$ equals $\sqrt{(a^2)}$; hence, the absolute value is never negative. The absolute value symbol is frequently used with the order relations, $<$, $>$, $\leq$, and $\geq$, in order to denote intervals. Thus, $|x| < a$, where $a$ is some positive number, denotes the *open interval* $-a < x < a$; whereas $|x| \leq a$ stands for the *closed interval* $-a \leq x \leq a$. An expression of the type $|x - b| < a$, where $a > 0$ and $b$ is any real number, means $-a < (x - b) < a$ or, equivalently, $b - a < x < b + a$, an interval of width $2a$ centered at $b$.

## Division by Zero

*Division by zero is not defined in mathematics*, hence, in expressions that are the quotients of two variables, the value of the denominator cannot be zero. This fact is well established in mathematics, yet in the pharmacological literature we find expressions written in such a way that this rule is not followed. For example, the velocity of an enzyme–substrate reaction is given by the Michaelis equation (see p.29)

$$V = \frac{V_{\max}[S]}{[S] + K}$$

where $[S]$ is the substrate concentration, and $V_{\max}$ and $K$ the constants. This equation is often written

$$V = \frac{V_{\max}}{1 + K/[S]}.$$

The latter form has no mathematical meaning at $[S] = 0$, whereas the former (correctly) gives the value $V = 0$ at $[S] = 0$.

## Errors and Significant Figures

Care must be exercised in the way we express the numbers that arise from measurement. The digits in a number that are needed to express the precision of the measurement from which the number was derived are known as *significant figures*. For example, if the dosage of some drug is reported as 2.54 mg/liter we understand that the precision used in giving the dose was such that the error was less than 0.005 mg/liter, that is, the dose $D$ is within the interval $2.535 < D < 2.545$. The number 2.54 contains *three significant* figures. If, however, the dose is expressed as 2.540 mg/liter, the notation implies an error less than 0.0005. Note that *final* zeros count as significant figures. A number such as 0.0015 has only *two significant* figures since the two zeros after the decimal point serve only to give the order of magnitude. The most frequent errors in notation arise in the measure of final zeros. One should avoid, for example, writing the speed of light as 186,000 miles/s, since this notation would mean that the speed is expressed with a precision of 1 mile/s. It would be better to write 186 thousand or $1.86 \times 10^5$ miles/s.

When arithmetic operations are performed on numbers that represent measured quantities, the errors may build to the extent that they are of some importance. The following rules are discussed in detail in books on numerical analysis and will serve as practical guides in the analysis of dose–response data:

1.  In addition and subtraction, we should retain in each number only as many figures to the right of the decimal point as there are in the number that contains the fewest such figures. For example, in adding the numbers (which might represent quantities of drug recovered in three separate extractions) $50.3 + 6.75 + 0.37529$, we should write $50.3 + 6.8 + 0.4$.

2.  In multiplication and division, we report the result with sufficient figures to express the precision of the *least* accurately known quantity. For example, $506.30 \times 7.2/5.88$, which might (incorrectly) be written 619.959 should be reported with 2 significant figures because the least accurately known number, 7.2, has 2 significant figures. Thus, we should write $6.2 \times 10^2$ for the result of these operations.

## Relations and Functions

The word *relation* is used to denote two sets of elements and a rule that as- sociates an element of the first set with an element of the second set. In particular, if one set consists of drug dosages, and the other set consists of the corresponding responses produced by those doses, we have a relation that we call a dose– response relation. What we have, then, is a set of *ordered pairs* $(D_1, E_1), (D_2, E_2)$, etc. In this definition there is no requirement that the effect produced by a given dose be unique. Indeed, in most cases in pharmacology we expect to get a range of effects for a given dose. In modern mathematics the term *function* is used to denote a relation in which there is a *unique* second element (effect) correspond- ing to each first element (dose). Since uniqueness is not the rule in pharmacology, it is technically incorrect to say that $E$ is a function of $D$. Nevertheless, the practice is widespread and, therefore, we shall use the term function even for these "multiple-valued" cases.

The two sets, $\{D_i\}$ and $\{E_i\}$, are called the *domain* and *range*, respectively. An element of the domain is often referred to as the *independent variable*, whereas an element in the range is termed the *dependent variable*. Thus, the drug dose is the independent variable, and the measured response is the de- pendent variable.

It is customary to represent functions by letters such as $f$, $g$, $F$, $\theta$, etc. If $D$ is an element of the domain of the function $f$, then the symbol "$f(D)$," read

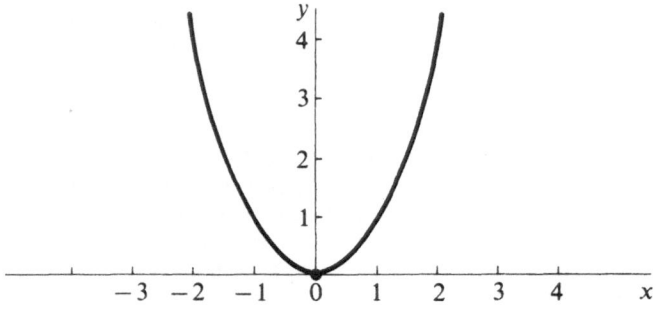

**Figure 2.1** The parabola $y = x^2$

"$f$ of $D$," is used to represent the corresponding element $E$ in the range. We write $E = f(D)$ and call the element $E$ or $f(D)$ the *value* of the function $f$ for the element $D$. In most mathematics textbooks, the symbols $x$ and $y$ are used for the elements in the domain and range, respectively. We will frequently use these symbols.

The ordered pairs $(x, y)$ of the function $f$ are often plotted as the rectangular (Cartesian) coordinates of a point in the $X$-$Y$ plane. The entire collection of such points constitutes the *graph* of the function. Thus, the graph of a function $f$ defined by the equation $y = f(x) = x^2$ contains points such as $(0, 0)$, $(1, 1)$, $(-1, 1)$, $(2, 4)$, $(-2, 4)$, $(1.5, 2.25)$, etc. This function consists of an infinite set of points. The second element of each pair $(y)$ is determined by substituting the value of the first element $(x)$ in the equation. For example, for the function $f$ above, the number paired with 1 is $1^2 = 1$; hence $(1, 1)$ is a point of the graph. The number paired with 2 is $2^2 = 4$, giving the point $(2, 4)$, etc. The domain of this function is the set of all real numbers. The range is the set of all nonnegative numbers. Its Cartesian graph, shown in Figure 2.1, is the familiar parabola. Figure 2.2 shows the Cartesian graphs of several types of functions that occur in pharmacology.

The functions illustrated in Figure 2.2 are described by equations. It is important to note that the equation is a statement only of the rule of correspondence between the variables $x$ and $y$, and, as such, it does not define the function. The domain ($x$'s) and the range ($y$'s) must be specified. Thus, a function $f$ defined by the equation $y = 2x + 5$, for *all* $x$, is not the same as the function given by $y = 2x + 5$ for a *limited domain*, say $-1 < x < 1$. In many applications, the domain and the range are limited. Hence, an equation may be a valid rule of correspondence only over some limited domain of definition. For example, a dose–response relation may be described in some situations by an equation of the form $y = ax/(x + b)$. It is clear, however, that the domain (the set of doses) is some finite set and, thus, a hyperbolic curve such as that of Figure 2.2c would not define the true dose–response relation; only a piece of the hyperbola, that between $x = 0$ and $x =$ the maximum dose, is applicable.

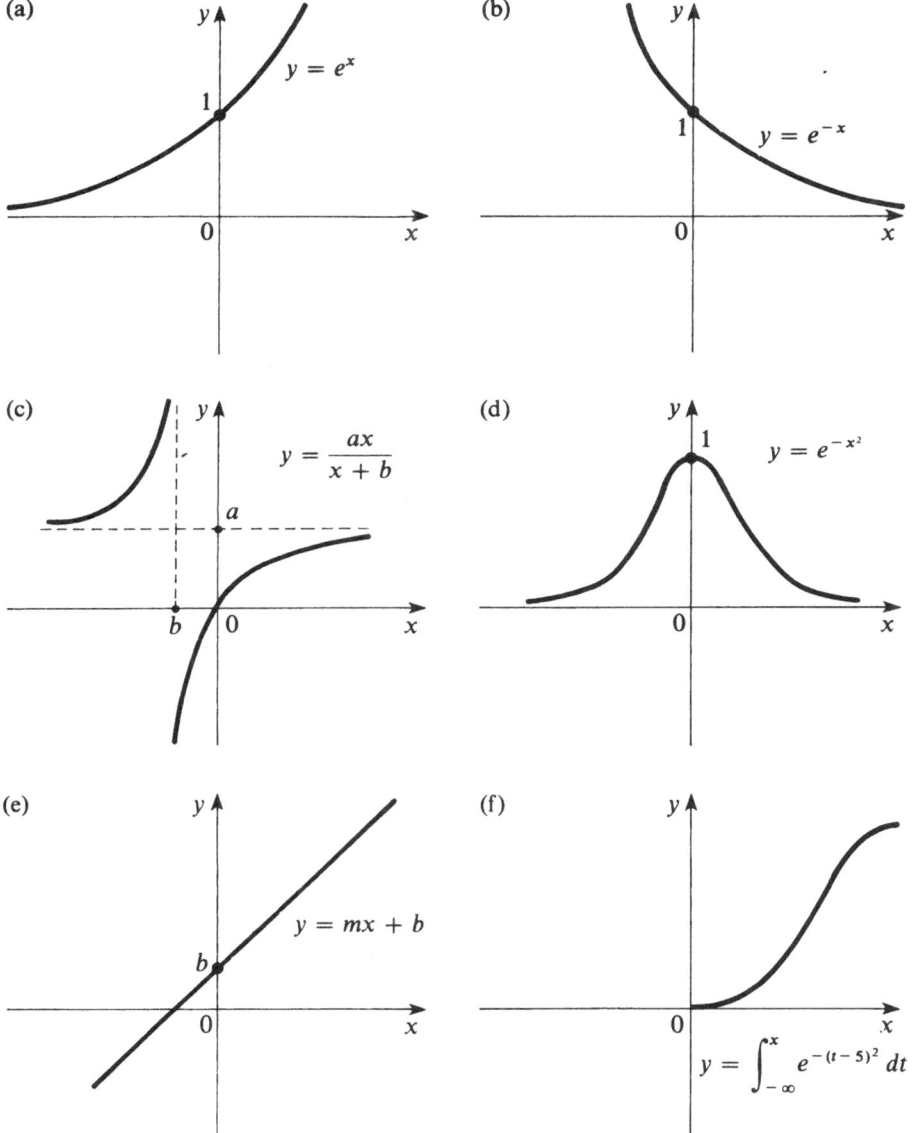

**Figure 2.2** Graphs of familiar functions.

## The Linear Function

One of the most important functions is the *linear function*, so called because its graph (in Cartesian coordinates) is a straight line. The equation of the linear function is

$$y = mx + b \tag{2.1}$$

where $m$ and $b$ are constants. Figure 2.3 shows the graphs of several different linear functions.

The number $m$, the coefficient of $x$, is the *slope* of the line. The slope is the ratio of the *rise* to the *run* and will be positive for lines that slant to the right and negative for lines that slant to the left. Of course, if $m = 0$, the line is horizontal. The number $b$ in the linear equation is the value of $y$ when $x = 0$; hence, $b$ is the Y-intercept. Thus, if $b = 0$, the graph of the linear equation passes through the origin. If the equation is given in the form $y = mx + b$ we can immediately recognize the slope and the Y-intercept. For example, $y = -5x + 3$ is the equation of a line of slope $= -5$ and Y-intercept $= +3$. Conversely, if we are given the values of the slope and the Y-intercept, we can immediately write the equation of the line. For example, a line of slope $+3$ and Y-intercept $-4$ has the equation $y = 3x - 4$.

Very often two variables $x$ and $y$ are *linearly related*, yet the equation of the relation may not be in the form $y = mx + b$. In such cases we can do some algebra in order to get the equation in the $(mx + b)$ form. For example, the equation $4x - 2y + 10 = 0$ can be transformed into $y = 2x + 5$ by transposition and division. The advantage of such a transformation is the instant recognition of the graph when we have *explicit* values of the slope and the

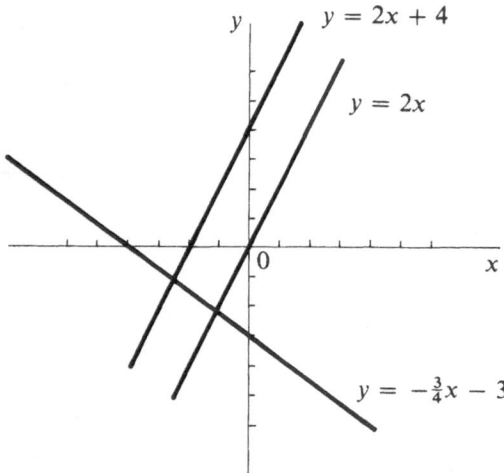

**Figure 2.3** Linear functions.

*Y*-intercept. Many graphical analyses of pharmacological data come down to a recognition of the slope and intercept of a line, as we will see in the next section. Hence, it is advisable to be thoroughly familiar with the linear function and to be able to recognize the slope and intercept from the equation.

When written in the form $y = mx + b$, the linear function is said to be in the *slope-intercept* form. It is convenient to have other forms. For example, suppose that we know the slope $m$ and one point $(x_1, y_1)$. It follows that we can substitute $x_1$ for $x$ and $y_1$ in Equation (2.1). Hence $y_1 = mx_1 + b$. Solving for $b$ gives $b = y_1 - mx_1$. If this expression for $b$ is inserted into Equation (2.1) we get, after rearrangement

$$y - y_1 = m(x - x_1). \tag{2.2}$$

Equation (2.2) is known as the *point-slope* form of the linear equation since the slope and the coordinates of one point can be instantly recognized from this form. Thus, $y - 5 = 3(x - 7)$ is a line of slope 3 that contains the point $(7, 5)$, while $y - 2 = -(x + 1)$ is a line of slope $-1$ that contains the point $(-1, 2)$. If this last example is not clear, the reader should note that the equation of this line can be written as $y - 2 = (-1)(x - [-1])$. The point-slope form is especially useful in the discussion of linear regression (see p. 98).

There are, of course, other forms for expressing the linear function. For our purposes, however, the two that we have discussed are sufficient. When the equation of the line is known, regardless of the form of the equation, all the information needed about the line can be obtained. For example, we might wish to know the value of the $x$-intercept. In that case we merely let $y = 0$ and solve for $x$. In several applications in the next section, we will have occasions to find the $x$-intercept of a line.

If the variables are related by the equation $y = mx$, the line passes through the origin. This special kind of linear function is called a *direct proportion*. Thus, when it is said that $y$ is directly proportional to $x$, the statement means that $y = mx$ for some number $m$. The number $m$ is referred to as the *proportionality constant*. Graphically, the proportionality constant is the slope of the line through the origin. An understanding of direct proportion is especially important in our subsequent applications, particularly when we discuss the theories of drug action in Chapter 3.

It is worth repeating that several graphical procedures used in pharmacology come down to an analysis of a linear relationship between two variables. Hence, the modest amount of mathematics contained in this section is absolutely essential to an understanding of these procedures.

An equation of the form $ax + by + c = 0$, where $a$, $b$, and $c$ are constants, with at least one of $a$ and $b$ not equal to zero, represents a straight line. Note that if $b \neq 0$ this form may be written $y = -(a/b)x - (c/b)$; thus the slope is $-a/b$ and the intercept is $-c/b$. If $b = 0$ the line is vertical. In this case the slope is not defined. The equation of a vertical line has the form $x = $ constant. Since every straight line, including a vertical line, may be written in the form $ax + by + c = 0$ for some choice of $a$, $b$, and $c$, this form is often referred to as the *general linear equation.*

## Equations in Linear Form: Scatchard and Lineweaver–Burk Plots

The equation $y = 2x^2 + 5$ is plotted in Figure 2.4. Clearly $y$ and $x$ are not linearly related, since the equation is not in the form $y = mx + b$. The graph is a parabola, a curve very different from a straight line. The equation can, however, be put into linear form if a *new variable* is introduced. Thus, let $u = x^2$, in which case the equation $y = 2x^2 + 5$ becomes $y = 2u + 5$. The relation between $y$ and $u$ is linear, whereas the relation between $y$ and $x$ is nonlinear. Figure 2.5 gives the graph of $y$ against $u$ or, equivalently, the graph of $y$ against $x^2$. It is seen, therefore, that by some suitable transformation we were able to put the equation into linear form. The graphs, though different in appearance, provide the same information about the relation between the variables $x$ and $y$. A graph is, of course, just a method of displaying the relation between the variables. Although in the most common graphing method we plot one variable ($y$) against the other ($x$), there are numerous situations in which there may be some good reason to plot $y$ against $x^2$, or $y$ against log $x$. The "good reason" is often the desire to display the relation as a straight line. This was the case in the previous example. Straight lines are convenient.

As another example, consider the equation $y = 2x/(x + 5)$, $(x \geq 0)$. The graph of this relation is shown in Figure 2.6. Let us now introduce new variables $v = 1/y$ and $u = 1/x$. Substitution of these into the equation $y = 2x/(x + 5)$

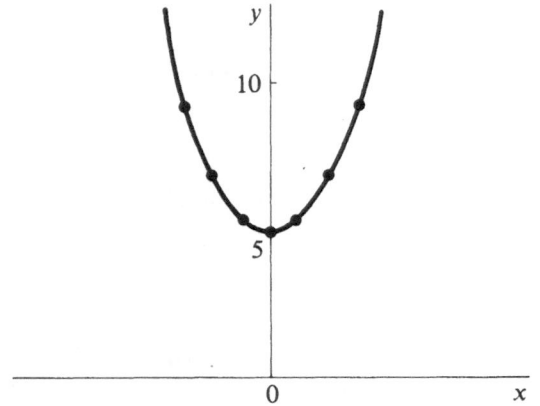

**Figure 2.4** Graph of $y = 2x^2 + 5$.

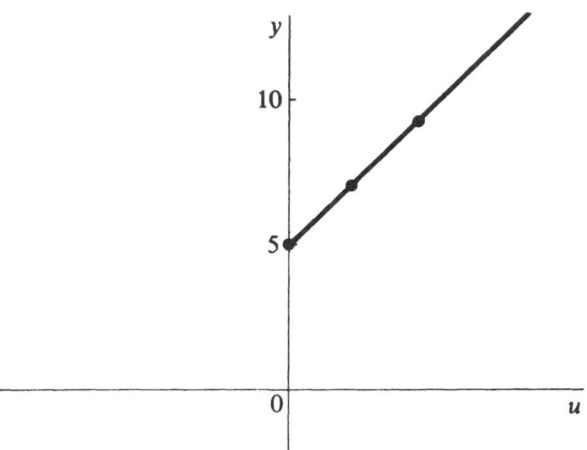

**Figure 2.5** Under the transformation $u = x^2$ the parabola of Figure 2.4 becomes the linear function $y = 2u + 5$.

yields $v = (5/2)u + 1/2$; thus $v$ and $u$ are linearly related. The graph of $v$ against $u$ is shown in Figure 2.7. The transformation $v = 1/y$, $u = 1/x$, produced in this case a straight line. This particular transformation is common in biochemistry and pharmacology as we shall see. The plot that results is referred to as a *double-reciprocal* plot. It should be noted that the double-reciprocal plot has no point corresponding to $x = 0$, $y = 0$, since division by zero is not defined.

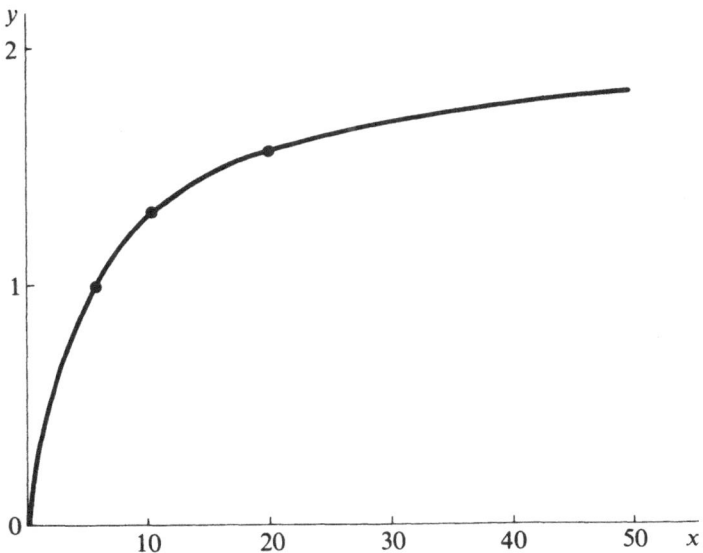

**Figure 2.6** The hyperbolic curve $y = 2x/(x + 5)$, $x \geq 0$.

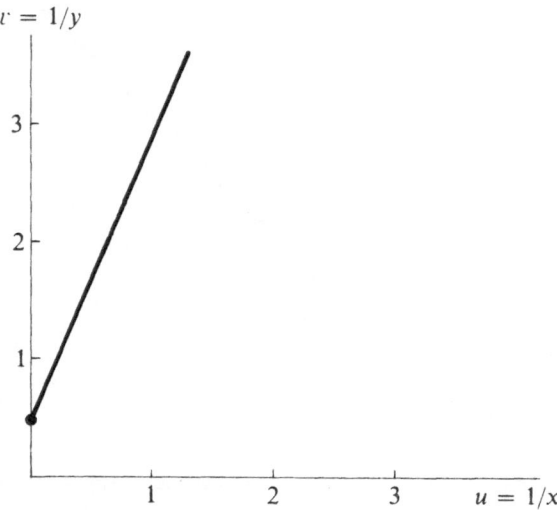

**Figure 2.7** Double-reciprocal plot of the hyperbola shown in Figure 2.6.

The previous examples serve only to remind the reader that there are other ways of plotting data.* The examples themselves have no other significance. We now discuss two graphical procedures which are actually used in pharmacology.

### The Scatchard Plot

Application of the law of mass action to the combination of a small molecule A with a protein R ($A + R \rightleftharpoons AR$) gives

$$\frac{[R][A]}{[RA]} = K \tag{2.3}$$

where $[R]$ and $[A]$ are the respective concentrations of unbound protein and reactant, $[RA]$ is the bound concentration, and $K$ is the equilibrium constant. Denoting the total protein concentration by $[R]_t$, it follows that $[R] = [R]_t - [RA]$. Thus, Equation (2.3) becomes

$$\frac{([R]_t - [RA])[A]}{[RA]} = K$$

or,

$$\frac{[RA]}{[A]} = -\frac{[RA]}{K} + \frac{[R]_t}{K}. \tag{2.4}$$

* A further discussion is given on page 38.

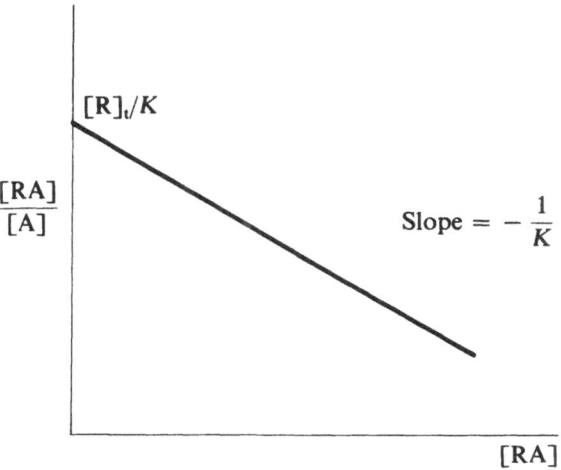

**Figure 2.8** Scatchard plot.

If we let $y = [RA]/[A]$ and $x = [RA]$, Equation (2.4) becomes

$$y = -\frac{1}{K}x + \frac{[R]_t}{K}.$$ 
(2.5)

Since $[R]_t$ and $K$ are constants, Equation (2.5) is linear with slope $-1/K$ and $y$-intercept $[R]_t/K$. The quantity $y$ is the ratio of bound to free substance, and this ratio is plotted against the bound concentration $x$, giving a theoretically linear plot in this case. This type of plot was used by Scatchard[3] in his study of the attractions of proteins for small molecules and ions (Fig. 2.8).

### The Lineweaver–Burk Plot

In the study of enzyme kinetics the enzyme E combines with substrate S to form a complex, ES. The rate of enzyme catalyzed reaction per unit volume, denoted by $V$, is related to the substrate concentration $[S]$ according to

$$V = \frac{V_{max}[S]}{[S] + K_m},$$ 
(2.6)

where $V_{max}$ is the maximum rate and $K_m$ is a constant. Equation (2.6) is usually attributed to Michaelis and Menten.[2] For practical applications, Equation (2.6) is transformed by taking reciprocals of both sides:

$$\frac{1}{V} = \frac{K_m}{V_{max}} \cdot \frac{1}{[S]} + \frac{1}{V_{max}}.$$ 
(2.6')

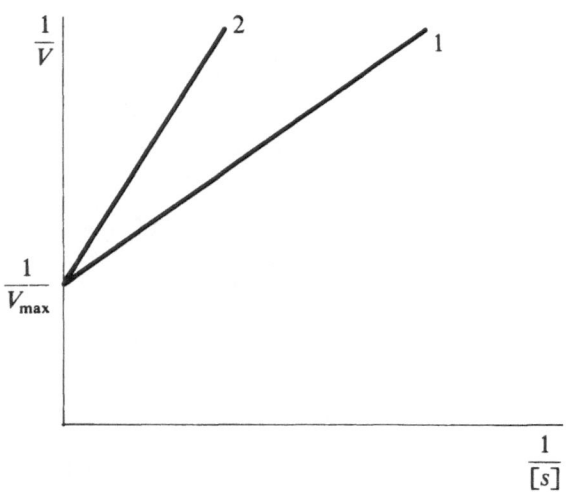

**Figure 2.9** Lineweaver–Burk plots. Curve 1: Substrate only; curve 2: the effect of a competitive inhibitor is to increase the slope.

Letting $y = 1/V$ and $x = 1/[S]$, we get

$$y = \frac{K_m}{V_{max}} x + \frac{1}{V_{max}}. \tag{2.7}$$

Since $K_m$ and $V_{max}$ are constants, Equation (2.8) is linear in $y$ and $x$ (or in $1/V$ and $1/[S]$). This type of plot, in which $1/V$ is plotted against $1/[S]$ is known as a Lineweaver–Burk plot and is a common method used to determine the constants $V_{max}$ and $K_m$. The $Y$-intercept gives $1/V_{max}$, whereas the slope gives $K_m/V_{max}$ from which $K_m$ is computed (Fig. 2.9).

An enzyme-catalyzed reaction may be inhibited by a second substance. In one type of inhibition, called *competitive inhibition*, the inhibitor molecule attaches itself to the enzyme at the site normally occupied by the substrate molecule. However, an excess of the substrate can completely restore the reaction rate. In other words, the antagonism is surmountable. The reaction rate in the presence of the competitive inhibitor in concentration $[I]$ is

$$V = \frac{V_{max}[S]}{[S] + K_m(1 + [I]/K_I)} \tag{2.8}$$

where $K_I$ is the dissociation constant of the inhibitor–enzyme complex. When placed in double-reciprocal form,

$$\frac{1}{V} = \frac{K_m}{V_{max}}\left(1 + \frac{[I]}{K_I}\right) \cdot \frac{1}{[S]} + \frac{1}{V_{max}} \tag{2.9}$$

a straight line is obtained as in the previous case. However, the slope is steeper by the factor $(1 + [I]/K_I)$ as seen in Figure 2.9. (See pages 56 and 66 for applications to dose–response data.)

## Power Functions

The linear equation is characterized by the fact that it has only first powers of $x$ and $y$. The reader is no doubt familiar with equations in which either $x$ or $y$ or both are raised to a power. The equations $y = x^2$, and $x^2 + y^2 = 1$, are examples of such *nonlinear* equations.

The equation

$$y = C_0 + C_1 x + C_2 x^2 + \cdots + C_n x^n \tag{2.10}$$

where $C_0, C_1, \ldots, C_n$ are constants and $n$ is a *positive integer*, is called a *polynomial*. Such equations are met early in the study of algebra because the computation of $y$ for any $x$ involves only the operations of addition and multiplication. (Raising a number to a positive integral power is just repeated multiplication.) Thus, $y = x^2$, and $y = 5 - x^3 + 10x^7$, are examples of polynomials. The linear function $y = b + mx$ is, of course, also a polynomial.

If $P(x)$ and $Q(x)$ are polynomials, a function of the form

$$y = \frac{P(x)}{Q(x)} \tag{2.11}$$

is called a *rational function*. For example, the function $y = ax/(b + x)$, discussed previously,* is a rational function. The evaluation of rational functions involves an additional arithmetic operation, namely, division. Of course, since division by zero is not defined, a rational function has no value at any $x$ for which the denominator polynomial vanishes. For example, the function $(x^2 + x)/(x - 2)$ has no value at $x = 2$. At such values of $x$ the function and, hence, its graph, is discontinuous (Fig. 2.10). A moment's reflection will convince the reader that all polynomials are special cases of rational functions.

With rational functions, we encounter powers of $x$ which are positive integers. Yet in both pure and applied mathematics, powers which are positive and negative fractions and irrational numbers are met. For example, the human body surface area has been empirically shown to depend on the height, $x$, raised to the power 0.725, and mathematics texts consider functions like $y = x^{-\pi}$. The interpretation of the power as the number of times $x$ is multiplied by itself is lost in such cases. The reader may recall that raising a number to a general power is attained from a collection of precise definitions beginning with $x^{1/n}$, where $x$ is a positive number and $n$ is a positive integer. We wish to preserve the rule that for any number $x$ and any pair of positive integers $m$ and $n$, $x^{m+n} = x^m x^n$. Thus we define $x^{1/n}$ to be a unique positive number $y$ such that $y^n = x$. This number $y$ is called the $n$th root of $x$. In the case in which $x = 0$, we define $x^{1/n}$ to be equal to 0.

---

* Equation (1.1) was of this form in terms of $E$ and $D$.

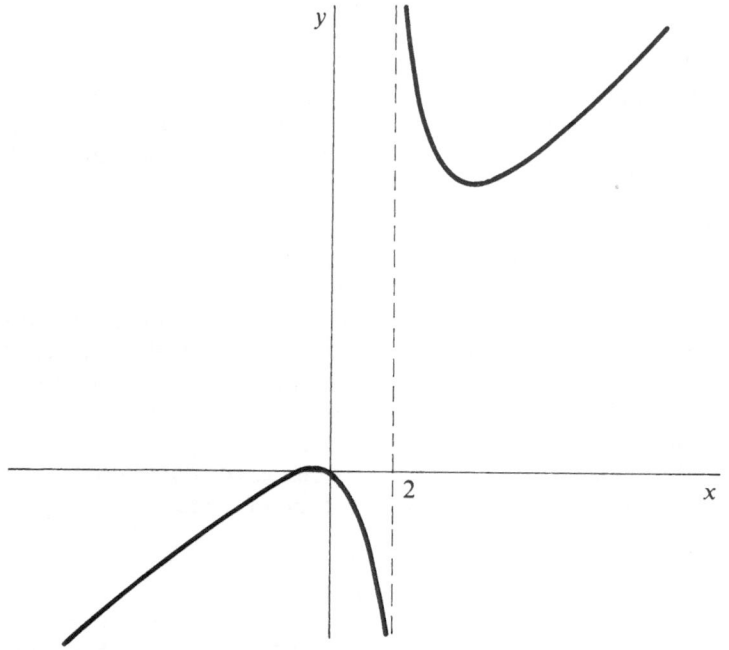

**Figure 2.10** Graph of $y = (x^2 + x)/(x - 2)$. The function is not defined at $x = 2$.

Having defined $x^{1/n}$ we can now define $x^{m/n}$, where $m$ and $n$ are positive integers:

$$x^{m/n} = (x^{1/n})^m = (x^m)^{1/n}. \qquad (2.12)$$

For *negative powers* (which may now be fractions) we define $x^{-P}$ to be equal to $1/x^P$, where $x > 0$ and $P$ is some positive fraction. Hence, $x^{-2/3} = 1/x^{2/3}$, and $x^{-5} = 1/x^5$. In order to preserve the rule that $x^{p+q} = x^p x^q$, we must *define $x^0$ to be equal to 1*, since $x^0 = x^{p-p} = x^p \cdot x^{-p} = x^p/x^p$.

The above definitions for $x^p$ when the power $p$ is a fraction (rational number), whether positive or negative, cover a lot of ground. However, these definitions do not include $x^p$ when $P$ is not a fraction. Hence, numbers such as $\sqrt{(2)}$, $\sqrt{(3)}$, $\pi$, $e$, ..., and any other *irrational number*, are not yet possible powers of $x$. Is a definition possible that would still preserve the rules $x^{p+q} = x^p x^q$, $x^0 = 1$, for irrational numbers $p$ and $q$? The answer, of course, is yes. The interested reader should consult a good calculus book for the details.*

---

* See references at the end of this chapter.

## Exponential Functions: Half-Life

In the previous section we defined $a^x$ for positive $a$ and rational $x$. We did not give a definition of $a^x$ for irrational $x$ but only mentioned that a definition was possible. For practical purposes it is sufficient to know that when $x$ is irrational, say $x = \pi$, $a^x$ can be approximated to any desired degree of accuracy by expressing $x$ (in this case $\pi$) to a sufficient number of decimal places. Thus, $a^\pi \approx a^{3.14}$ or, if more accuracy is needed, $a^\pi \approx a^{3.1416}$. Note that 3.14 and 3.1416 are *rational* numbers which *approximate* $\pi$. In what follows, therefore, we will assume that it is possible to discuss $a^x$ for positive $a$ and any *real value* of $x$.

The function $y = b^x$ ($b > 0$) is called an *exponential function* with base $b$. The domain of this function is the set of real numbers. Its range is the set $0 < y < \infty$ (all positive numbers). The usual "laws of exponents" hold for this function for $a > 0$ and $b > 0$:

$$\begin{aligned} b^x \cdot b^y &= b^{x+y} \\ (b^x)^y &= b^{xy} \\ (ab)^x &= a^x \cdot b^x \\ b^0 &= 1 \end{aligned} \tag{2.13}$$

Although the choice of base $b$ can be any positive number, for practical purposes $b$ is taken to be a number greater than one. With $b > 1$ the function $y = b^x$ is *monotone increasing*. Graphically, this means that $y$ increases as $x$ increases. The number $b$ that is most important is the irrational number "$e$" which is approximately equal to the rational number 2.71828. The importance of the number $e$ is intimately tied to concepts involving calculus. In many applications the function defined by $y = e^x$ arises. An alternate notation for this function is $y = \exp(x)$. Values of $\exp(x)$ appear in tables* and are available from many modern electronic calculators. The graph of $y = \exp(x)$ is shown in Figure 2.11, along with $y = \exp(-x)$, a monotone *decreasing* function.

Functions of the form $y = Ae^{-bx}$ arise in many applications. For example, $y$ might represent the amount of drug in plasma at time $x$. The number $b$ is related to the rate of disappearance. Graphs of functions of this type are shown in Figure 2.12 for several different values of $b$. The reciprocal of $b$ is called the *time constant*. The number $\ln(2)/b$ is called the *half-life* [see also Equation (2.24)]. Figure 2.13 illustrates an important property of the exponential function $y = Ae^{-bx}$. As $x$ goes from 0 to some value $a$, the value of $y$ decreases from $A$ to some fraction of $A$, specifically $e^{-ba}(A)$. We denote $e^{-ba}$ by $f$. Now as $x$ goes from $a$ to $2a$, $y$ is decreased to $Ae^{-b(2a)} = A(e^{-ba})^2 = Af^2$. Thus, as $x$ is incremented by the constant amount $a$, the value of $y$ is decreased to $f$ times the value it had at the

---

* See appendix Table A.6.

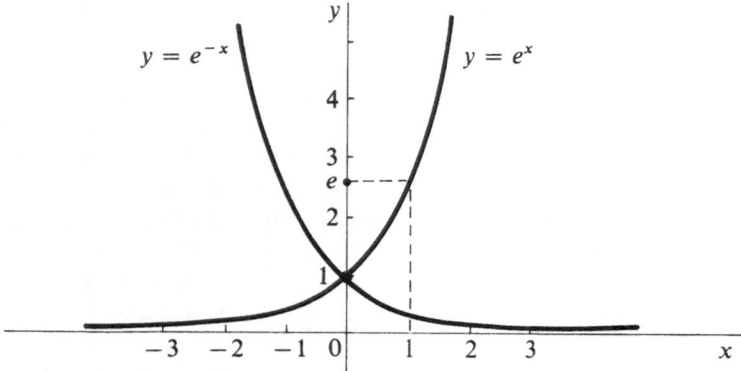

**Figure 2.11** Exponential functions.

beginning of the increment. In particular, if $f = 1/2$ then $a$ is the familiar *half-life* of the exponential function. It should be noted that the half life is meaningful only for an exponential function. In general, other decreasing functions do not have this property. Of course, the increasing exponential, $y = Ae^{bx}$, $(b > 0)$ will have the property of increasing to a constant factor

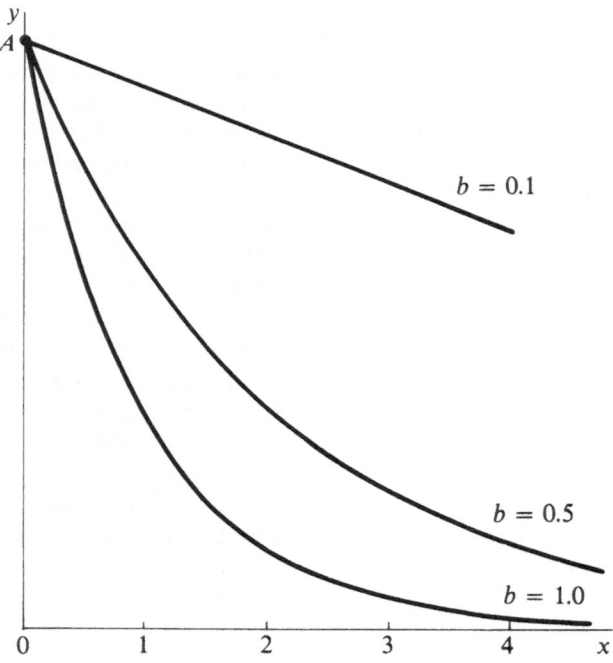

**Figure 2.12** The function $y = Ae^{-bx}$ for several values of $b$.

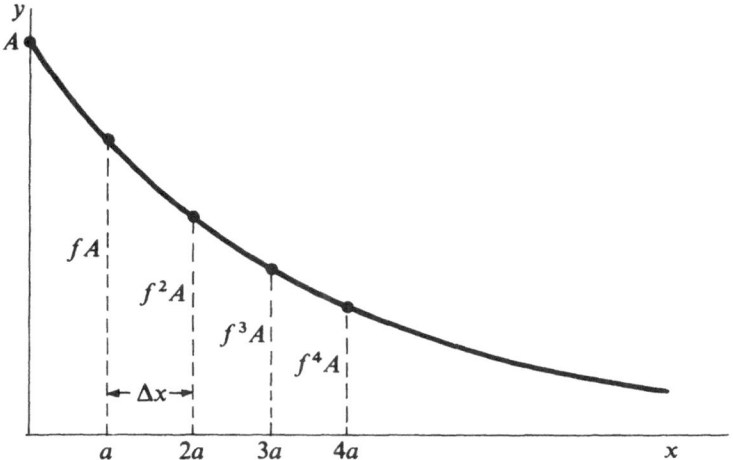

**Figure 2.13** A constant increment $\Delta x = a$ results in the same fractional decrease $f$ in $y$.

times $A$ whenever $x$ is incremented by a constant amount. Thus, one can talk about doubling times, tripling times, etc.

### Multiple Intravenous Injections

If some amount $I$ of drug is administered intravenously at equal time intervals $t_1, 2t_1, 3t_1, \ldots, nt_1$, for an indefinite time, will the amount in the plasma increase indefinitely, or will it stay less than some upper limit? The answer depends

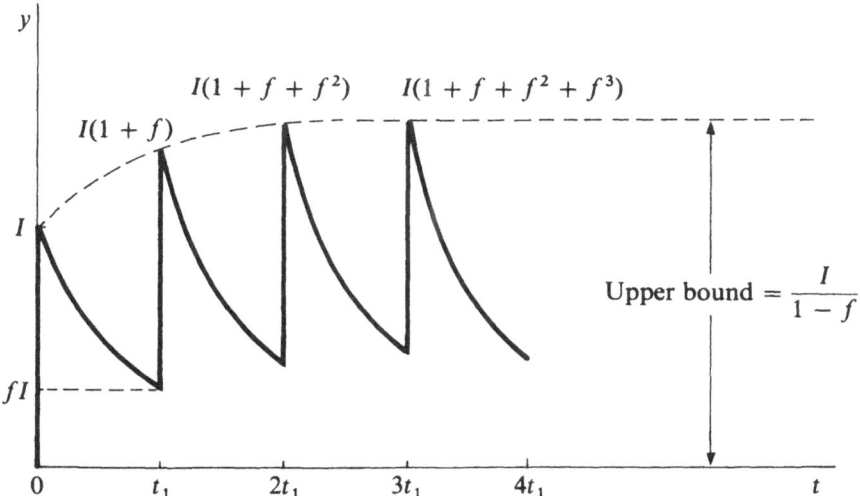

**Figure 2.14** Multiple intravenous injections.

upon the kinetics governing the elimination from the plasma. If the elimination is exponential, i.e., if the amount $y$ is related to dose $I$ and time $t$ according to

$$y = Ie^{-bt}, \tag{2.14}$$

then there is an *upper bound* to $y$, as we now show.

At time $t_1$, $y = Ie^{-bt_1}$. If we denote $e^{-bt_1}$ by $f$, then at time $t_1$, $y = If$. A second dose $I$ is given, bringing the total drug to $I + If$ or $I(1 + f)$. *This amount* now decays to a fraction $f$ of the amount during the interval $t_1$ to $2t_1$. Hence, at $t = 2t_1$, the amount is $f(I[1 + f]) = I(f + f^2)$. But a third dose is given instantly, bringing the total to $I + I(f + f^2)$ or $I(1 + f + f^2)$. If this process is continued indefinitely, the peaks (Fig. 2.14) are given by the *series* $I(1 + f + f^2 + f^3 + \cdots)$. As $f < 1$, the series *converges* to $I/(1 - f)$. Hence, the peaks, though increasing, *remain less than* $I/(1 - f)$. For example, if the time interval between doses is the half-life, then $f = \frac{1}{2}$ and the upper limit is $I/(1 - \frac{1}{2}) = 2I$. In deriving this expression we made use of the property of exponentials previously referred to. If the elimination were at a *constant* rate, rather than exponential, the peaks would have *no upper limit*.

Functions involving exponentials are common in pharmacology, especially in models describing the time course of drug concentration. For example, the drug concentration $C$ in some tissue compartment of volume $V$ depends upon the blood flow $Q$ to the tissue and the concentration in arterial blood $C_A$ according to

$$C = C_A(1 - e^{-(Q/V)t}) \tag{2.15}$$

whose graph is given in Figure 2.15.

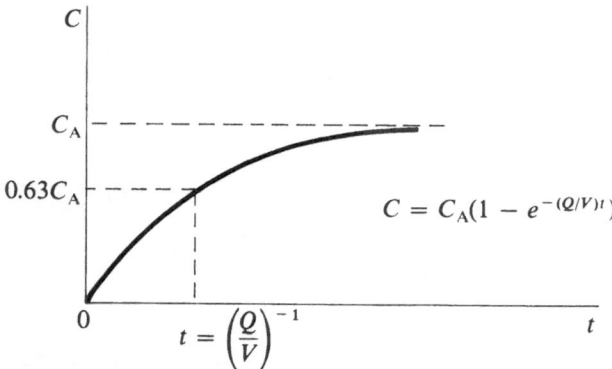

**Figure 2.15** Drug concentration $C$ in a tissue. $C_A$ is the concentration in arterial blood. At time $t = (Q/V)^{-1}$ the concentration is approximately 63% of $C_A$.

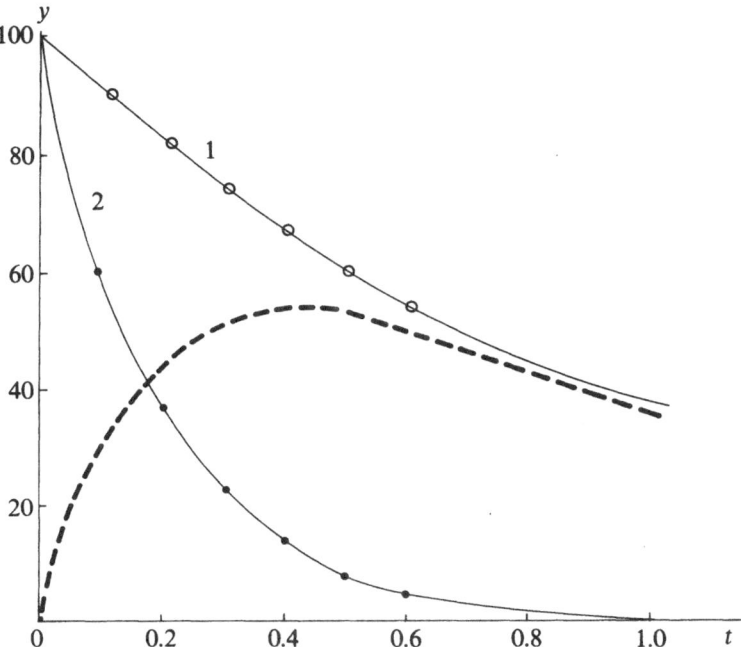

**Figure 2.16** Graph of $y = 100$ $(e^{-t} - e^{-5t})$ shown as broken curve and plotted by subtracting the ordinates of curves 1 and 2. (Curve 1) $y = 100e^{-t}$; (curve 2) $y = 100e^{-5t}$.

As another example, if a single intravenous dose is given in a *two-compartment open model*,* one compartment being the plasma and the other some tissue, then the concentration in the tissue is given by an equation of the form

$$y = Ae^{-at} - Be^{-bt}. \tag{2.16}$$

(The significance of the constants $A$, $a$, $B$, and $b$ is discussed in Chapter 5.) A special case of Equation (2.16) is shown in Figure 2.16 in which the terms are graphed separately and then the *ordinates added* (algebraically) to give the composite graph of $y$ against $t$.

Finally, we should like to point out that functions which are sums (or differences) of even three exponentials may be encountered. Thus, a function of the form

$$y = Ae^{-at} + Be^{-bt} + Ce^{-ct} \tag{2.17}$$

has been shown to describe the brain concentration of morphine in the rat following a single intravenous injection.[1]

---

* See Equation (5.12) in Chapter 5.

When the equation is completely specified, i.e., when all the constants are known, the graphs are readily drawn. It takes a lot more labor to find the constants of the equation which "best" fits data derived from an experimental procedure. Rather tedious graphical methods have been used for this purpose[4] although sophisticated "curve fitting" subroutines are now accomplished more quickly with modern electronic computers.

## Logarithms and Logarithmic Functions: The Henderson–Hasselbach Equation

We saw that $b^p$ could be defined for any real number $p$ and $b > 0$. Let us consider $b^y$ for $b > 1$, and call its value $x$; i.e., $x = b^y$. Then $y$ *is called the logarithm of* $x$ *to the base* $b$ *and is written* $y = \log_b x$. Thus, $\log_{10} 10 = 1$, $\log_{10} 100 = 2$, and $\log_{10} 1000 = 3$, whereas $\log_{10} 10^{-1} = -1$, $\log_{10} 10^{-2} = -2$, etc. These cases, in which the base $b$ is taken to be 10, are very often used in pharmacology as well as in other branches of science. The number $e$ is also used since it is very convenient for theoretical purposes. Logarithms to the base 10 are called "common" logarithms, whereas those to the base $e$ are called "natural" logarithms. When no base is written, the common logarithm of a number $x$ will be denoted $\log x$, whereas the natural logarithm of $x$ will be denoted $\ln x$. Tables of both common and natural logarithms are numerous.* Also, many electronic calculators will give the natural or the common logarithm of any positive number. It should be noted that since $b^y > 0$, the logarithms of *negative numbers and the logarithm of zero are not defined here*. Since the expression $y = \log_b x$ is equivalent to $x = b^y$, we can substitute for $y$ in the exponent; hence

$$x = b^{\log_b x}. \tag{2.18}$$

Equation (2.18) is an identity which, of course, defines the logarithm.

The following properties of logarithms arise directly from the definition and the rules of exponents:

$$\begin{aligned}
\log_b xy &= \log_b x + \log_b y, \\
\log_b y/x &= \log_b y - \log_b x, \\
\log_b x^y &= y \log_b x.
\end{aligned} \tag{2.19}$$

The graph of the logarithmic function, $y = \log_b x$, $(b > 1)$ is shown in Figure 2.17. Note that $y$ increases as $x$ increases.

* Brief tables are contained in the appendix.

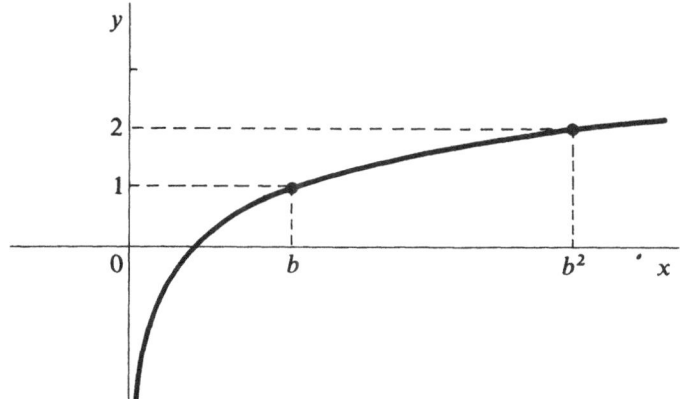

**Figure 2.17** The logarithmic function $y = \log_b x$.

The logarithm of a number is important in many applications. We have seen that "dose–response" data are often expressed as "log(dose)–response" data (see p. 7). Also, the familiar definition of $pH$ uses the logarithm: $pH = -\log[H^+]$, where $[H^+]$ is the concentration of hydrogen ion. Further, the widely used term "$pA_2$" for an antagonist drug is defined in terms of the logarithm: $pA_2 = -\log K_B$, where $K_B$ is the dissociation constant in the reaction between *antagonist* and receptor (see p. 62).

When we know the logarithm of a number $x$ to base $b$, we can find the logarithm of $x$ to *some other base a* by the conversion formula

$$\log_a x = \log_b x \cdot \log_a b. \qquad (2.20)$$

Such conversions frequently are made between bases 10 and $e$. From Equation (2.20)

$$\log_{10} x = \log_e x \cdot \log_{10} e \approx 0.434 \log_e x \qquad (2.21)$$

and

$$\log_e x = \log_{10} x \cdot \log_e 10 \approx 2.30 \log_{10} x. \qquad (2.22)$$

When we deal with exponential functions, such as $y = Ae^{-at}$, the use of logarithms permits a solution for $t$ in terms of $y$ as shown below:

$$y = Ae^{-at}$$

$$\ln y = \ln(A \cdot e^{-at}) = \ln A + \ln e^{-at}$$

$$\ln y = \ln A - at.$$

$$t = \frac{(\ln A - \ln y)}{a} = \frac{\ln(A/y)}{a}. \qquad (2.23)$$

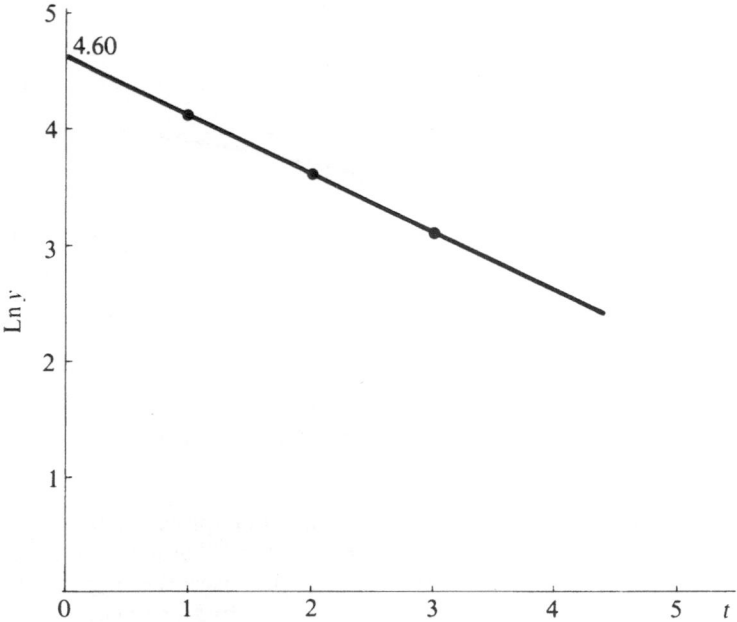

**Figure 2.18** Ln $y$ versus $t$ for the equation $y = 100e^{-0.5t}$.

In particular, we can get an explicit expression for the *half-life* of a decreasing exponential $y = Ae^{-at}$. By definition, the half-life is that value of $t$ for which $y = A/2$. Thus, from Equation (2.23)

$$t_{1/2} = \frac{\ln(2)}{a} \tag{2.24}$$

$$t_{1/2} \approx \frac{0.693}{a}. \tag{2.25}$$

Equations in linear form were discussed previously. Exponential functions are often put into linear form with the use of logarithms. For example, consider the decreasing exponential discussed previously, namely, $y = Ae^{-at}$. Taking logarithms gives

$$\ln y = \ln A - \ln e^{-at}$$
$$\ln y = \ln A - at. \tag{2.26}$$

Equation (2.26) is in *linear form*. The graph of $\ln y$ against $t$ is a straight line of slope $-a$ and $y$-intercept $\ln A$ as shown in Figure 2.18. This transformation is particularly useful when the data have an "exponential trend" but do not "fit" perfectly. In such cases plotting $\ln y$ against $t$ will produce a set of points that are approximately linear (Fig. 2.19). A straight line may then be drawn

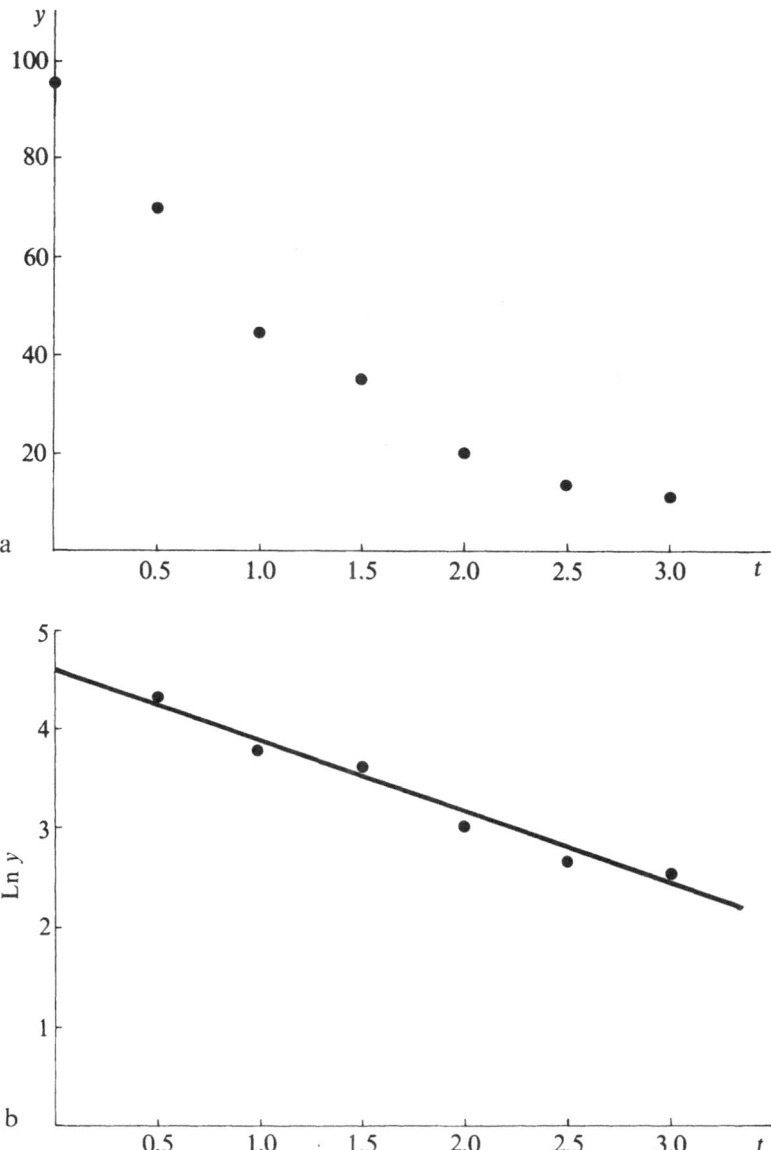

**Figure 2.19** (a) The set of points $(y, t)$; (b) consists of the points (Ln $y$, $t$) and displays a "linear trend."

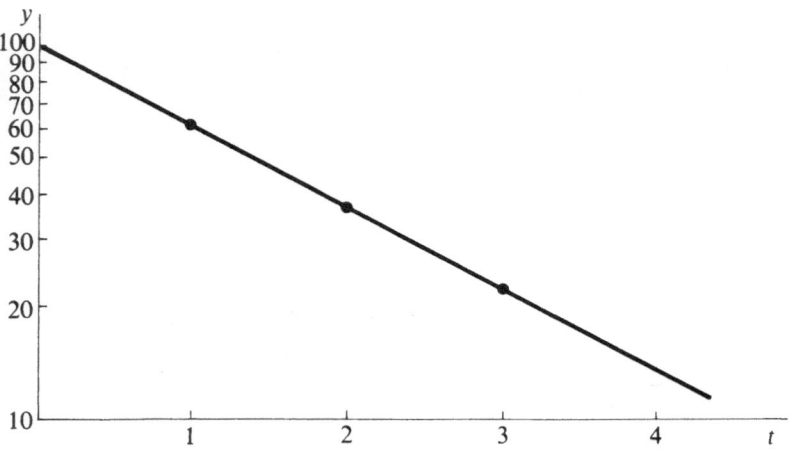

**Figure 2.20** The equation $y = 100e^{-0.5t}$ is plotted on semi-logarithmic graph paper.

which provides a good fit to the points. (See Chapter 4 for a discussion of techniques of curve fitting.) The line contains all the information needed to describe the exponential equation. Prepared graph paper having one scale calibrated logarithmically is convenient since the values are plotted directly and the resulting graph is linear as in Figure 2.20.

### The Henderson–Hasselbach Equation

The properties of logarithms are used in the derivation of the Henderson–Hasselbach equation. Recall that an acid HB dissociates to a proton $H^+$ and a base B. Thus,

$$HB \rightleftharpoons H^+ + B.$$

The equilibrium constant $K = k_1/k_2$ is given as

$$K = \frac{(H)(B)}{(HB)}.$$

Hence

$$\log K = \log(H) + \log(B) - \log(HB)$$

or

$$-\log(H) = -\log(K) + \log\frac{(B)}{(HB)}.$$

Denoting $-\log(H)$ by $pH$ and $-\log K$ by $pK$,

$$pH = pK + \log\frac{[B]}{[HB]}. \tag{2.27}$$

Equation (2.27) is the Henderson–Hasselbach equation. Its importance is related to the determination of the ratio of ionized to un-ionized forms of drugs.

For drugs that are weak acids the proton donor HB is in the un-ionized form. Thus, for such acids the Henderson–Hasselbach equation is $pH = pK + \log(\text{ionized/un-ionized})$. For weak bases (proton acceptors) the proton acceptor is un-ionized and, $pH = pK + \log(\text{un-ionized/ionized})$. Lipid membranes are relatively impermeable to the ionized forms of weak acids and bases. Suppose, for example, that a weak acid of $pK$ 4 is placed in gastric juice of pH 3. Substitution into the equation gives $3 = 4 + \log(\text{ionized/un-ionized})$; hence, the ratio of ionized to un-ionized $= 10^{-1}$. A weak base of $pK_4 = 4$ in this same medium gives (un-ionized/ionized) $= 10^{-1}$, that is, the base is more highly ionized than is the acid. Weak acids, therefore, are well absorbed from the stomach, whereas weak bases are poorly absorbed.

## Rate of Change and Drug Action

The rate of change of a function is an important concept in pharmacology. For example, let $x$ represent the concentration of drug in some compartment, and let $t$ represent the time. If at time $t = t_1$ the concentration of drug is $x_1$, and at some later time $t = t_2$ the concentration of drug is $x_2$, then the ratio

$$\frac{x_2 - x_1}{t_2 - t_1}$$

is a measure of the *rate* of change of concentration over the time interval $t_1$ to $t_2$. The *instantaneous rate of change* at time $t = t_1$ is the *limit* of the above ratio as $t_2$ approaches $t_1$. In other words, we select a time $t_2$ and measure the quantity $x_2$; then we examine the ratio $(x_2 - x_1)/(t_2 - t_1)$ as $t_2$ is taken closer and closer to $t_1$. If these ratios approach a value we call this instantaneous rate of change the *derivative* of $x$ with respect to t at $t_1$. Common notations for the derivative with respect to t are "$dx/dt$" and $x'(t)$. With reference to the graph of $x$ against $t$, the derivative is the *slope of the tangent* line $T$ at $t_1$ (Fig. 2.21). The slope of line $S$ is $(x_2 - x_1)/(t_2 - t_1)$ and represents the *average* rate of change over the interval $t_1$ to $t_2$.

The derivative at a particular value of $t$ is, of course, a number; hence, at every value of $t$ for which the derivative exists we get the value of the derivative. Thus, there is a correspondence between the set of times and the set of derivatives. In other words, the derivative of a function is also a function. If we denote by $f$ the function between $x$ and $t$, the derivative function is usually denoted by $f'$. We write, therefore, for the function $x = f(t)$

$$x' = f'(t)$$

or

$$\frac{dx}{dt} = f'(t).$$

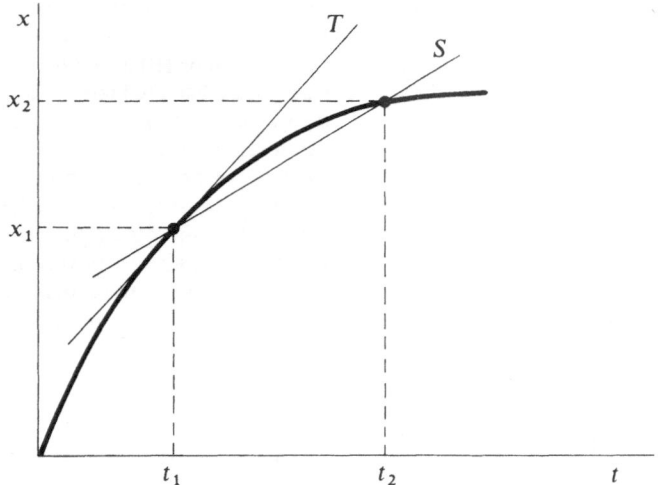

**Figure 2.21** The derivative is the slope of the tangent line $T$.

The rate of change procedure defining the derivative may be expressed formally for the function $x = f(t)$. The time interval is denoted "$\Delta t$." Thus, the increment in $x$ is $f(t + \Delta t) - f(t)$ and the average rate of change over the interval from $t$ to $t + \Delta t$ is

$$\frac{f(t + \Delta t) - f(t)}{\Delta t}.$$

The *limit* of this quotient as the increment $\Delta t$ becomes smaller and smaller is the derivative $f'(t)$:

$$f'(t) = \lim_{\Delta t \to 0} \frac{f(t + \Delta t) - f(t)}{\Delta t}. \tag{2.28}$$

Although our example used time $t$ as the independent variable, the derivative is similarly defined for functions involving any pair of variables such as $y$ and $x$. For example, $y$ could represent the measure of effect produced by a drug dose $x$. In general, the derivative $f'(x)$ or $dy/dx$ gives the rate of change of $y$ with respect to $x$ at some value $x$.

The most familiar examples of rates arise in physics as velocity and acceleration. *Velocity is the rate of change of position (or distance) with respect to time; acceleration is rate of change of velocity with respect to time.*

The process of obtaining the derivative is called *differentiation*. If one differentiates the derivative of a function $y = f(x)$ the new function is called the *second derivative*, denoted $f''(x)$. Thus, $f''(x) = df'(x)/dx$. Higher derivatives arise from repetition of this process. For example, the third derivative, $f'''(x)$, is the derivative of the second derivative, etc.

Rules for differentiating functions defined by equations may be found in numerous books dealing with differential calculus; some rules are given in Appendix C. Our interest is in the application of the derivative to models of drug action. For example, the kinetics which govern the passage of a drug from a biological compartment may be expressed in terms of the time derivative of drug concentration. Specifically, suppose that a certain drug leaves a body compartment (such as blood plasma) at a *constant rate c*. Denoting the quantity of drug in the compartment by $y$, we express the rate as the time derivative $dy/dt$ and, thus

$$\frac{dy}{dt} = -c \qquad (2.29)$$

is the mathematical description of the process. If, however, the *rate is directly proportional to the quantity of drug*, then

$$\frac{dy}{dt} = -ky \qquad (2.30)$$

is the appropriate mathematical description.*

As another example, let us consider the rate with which a chemical reaction, $A + B \to C$, takes place. The rate in this case refers to the rate of formation of product C. If, at some instant $t$, we denote by $x$ the number of moles of C that has been formed, then the rate of formation of C is $dx/dt$. Further, suppose that this *rate is proportional to the product of the available reactants*. If at the beginning ($t = 0$) the amounts of A and B are $A_0$ and $B_0$, respectively, then at a time at which $x$ moles of product have been formed, the molar quantities of the reactants are $(A_0 - x)$ and $(B_0 - x)$; hence

$$\frac{dx}{dt} = k(A_0 - x)(B_0 - x) \qquad (2.31)$$

is the equation for the reaction, where $k$ is the proportionality constant.

In each of these examples the derivative of a quantity arises naturally since the process is expressed as the rate of change of the quantity. Further mathematical operations are necessary in order to express the relationship between the variables in a way that does *not involve the derivative*. The fundamental operation needed is called *integration*.

---

* This type of elimination is called "first order." The constant $k$ is the "rate constant." Equation (2.29) describes a "zero order" process.

## Integration

In the previous section, we saw how problems are mathematically described as equations that involve the rate of change or derivative of a variable. An equation that involves the derivative is called a *differential equation*. Thus, we might have $dy/dx = x$. Here we are given that $y$ is a function of $x$ whose derivative is equal to $x$; we wish to express $y$ as a function of $x$. Any function of the form $y = x^2/2 + c$, where $c$ is a constant, will *satisfy* the differential equation. Hence, $y = \frac{1}{2}x^2 + c$ is the *solution* of the differential equation. The function $\frac{1}{2}x^2 + c$ is the *antiderivative* of $x$.

More generally, if the right side of the differential equation is a function $f(x)$, i.e., if $dy/dx = f(x)$, the solution is $y =$ the antiderivative of $f(x)$, denoted $\int f(x)dx$. The antiderivative is a function having the derivative $f(x)$. Finding the antiderivative of $f(x)$ may be difficult; it may even be impossible in the sense that there is *no known function* whose derivative is $f(x)$. When a real problem leads to one of these situations, approximate methods are applied.

A differential equation can, of course, have a right-hand side that involves $y$. [We saw this in our discussion of drug elimination, Equation (2.30).] For now we avoid discussing this situation and turn to a seemingly unrelated problem, that of finding areas.

Consider the continuous curve given by $y = f(x)$ shown in Figure 2.22. It is desired to find the area included between the curve, the $x$-axis and the two vertical lines at $x = a$ and $x = b$.

The approach we will take (and this is only one approach) is to cut the region into $n$ parallel vertical strips of equal width, treating these strips as rectangles by disregarding the "triangular regions" shown shaded in the figure. Then we will add the areas of these rectangles, called the sum $S_n$, and then evaluate the *limit of the sum* as the number of rectangles increases without bound ($n \to \infty$).

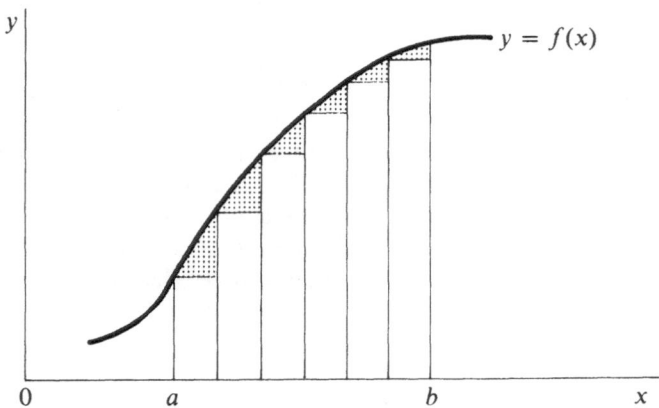

**Figure 2.22** Approximating the area under the curve.

The evaluation of this limit by direct calculation is surely a great deal of work, even for rather simple functions. *The fundamental theorem of the calculus* provides a method for finding the limit of this sum. We now describe the method.

First find the antiderivative $\int f(x)dx$, which we will denote by $F(x)$. Next, substitute $a$ and $b$ for $x$ in the antiderivative, getting $F(a)$ and $F(b)$, respectively. Then subtract $F(a)$ from $F(b)$; the difference is the required limit (or area):

$$\text{area} = \lim_{n \to \infty} S_n = F(b) - F(a). \qquad (2.32)$$

The common notation for the limit defining the area is $\int_a^b f(x)dx$; hence,

$$\int_a^b f(x)dx = F(b) - F(a). \qquad (2.33)$$

The limit defining the sum is an example of a *definite integral*, or "integral" for short. Geometrically the definite integral is the area under the curve $y = f(x)$ as shown in Figure 2.22, however, in a rigorous discussion of the definite integral the geometric interpretation is unnecessary. The fundamental theorem connects the derivative and the integral. Because of this connection, the antiderivative $\int f(x)dx = F(x)$ is called an *indefinite integral*, and the process of finding the antiderivative is called *integration*.

The case in which the derivative of a quantity is proportional to the quantity is of particular interest in pharmacology. For example, from Equation (2.30) $dy/dt = -ky$ where $k$ is a positive constant, arises in the passage of a drug from a body compartment; the variable $y$ stands for the quantity of drug at time $t$. (This same equation also describes the *decay* of radioactive substances.) The solution is the *decreasing* exponential function

$$y = y_0 e^{-kt}. \qquad (2.34)$$

From Equation (2.34) it is seen that $y_0$ is the value of $y$ at time $t = 0$.

A simple *growth process* is described by a differential equation similar to Equation (2.35), but without the minus sign, $dy/dt = ky$ ($k > 0$). The solution is the *increasing* exponential

$$y = y_0 e^{kt} \qquad (2.35)$$

in which $y_0$ is again the value of $y$ at $t = 0$.

Differential equations also arise in the study of drug–receptor interactions (see Chap. 3). The techniques for solving these equations are rather standard and the details may be found in texts which deal with the subject.* The solutions always involve the operation of integration.

---

* A brief discussion of methods for solving certain kinds of differential equations is presented in the appendix dealing with calculus.

## References

1. Dahlstrom, B. E., and Paalzow, L. K.: J. Pharmacokin. Biopharm., *3*:293, 1975.
2. Michaelis, L., and Menten, M. L.: Biochem. Z., *49*:333, 1913.
3. Scatchard, G.: Ann. N.Y. Acad. Sci., *51*:660, 1949.
4. Solomon, A. K.: in *Mineral Metabolism* I, part A, (Comar, C. L., and Bronner, F. eds.) New York, Academic Press, 1960, p. 119.

## Additional Readings

Batschelet, E. *Introduction to Mathematics for Life Scientists.* New York, Springer-Verlag, 1973.

Crowe, A., and Crowe, A. *Mathematics for Biologists.* London, Academic Press, 1969.

Franklin, D. A., and Newman, G. B. *A Guide to Medical Mathematics.* New York, John Wiley, 1973.

Grossman, S. I., and Turner, J. E. *Mathematics for the Biological Sciences.* New York, Macmillan, 1974.

Rainville, E. D. *Elementary Differential Equations.* 5th ed. New York, Macmillan, 1974.

Rubinow, S. I. *Introduction to Mathematical Biology.* New York, John Wiley, 1975.

Thomas, G. B. *Calculus and Analytic Geometry,* 5th ed. Reading, Mass., Addison-Wesley, 1979.

# Kinetics of Drug–Receptor Interaction: Interpreting Dose–Response Data

## Chapter 3

### Pharmacological Receptor

The concept of the pharmacological receptor was introduced by Langley[28] and by Ehrlich.[11] Langley's formulation was based on experiments in which he applied nicotine to small regions of a muscle surface. He observed that a muscle twitch occurred only when the nicotine was applied to certain small areas of the muscle surface and, hence, he postulated the existence of a *receptive substance* at those small areas. Ehrlich, on the other hand, worked with various dyes, observing that some cells were stained more deeply or in a different way from other cells. These observations suggested to Ehrlich that a general theory could be developed that would explain the *selective action* of drugs. Much study since then, particularly studies that showed that other substances could inhibit or block the specific action of a drug, have given general acceptance to the receptor concept. The most general definition of a receptor is that it is *that component of the cell that combines chemically with a drug in order to produce an effect*. For the most part we know little about the chemical or physico-chemical makeup of the receptor. In that respect, the receptor has been described as a measure of our ignorance by Gero[20]; yet the concept has proved most helpful in pharmacology.

There is much about drugs and receptors that is similar to substrates and enzymes. In the study of both we apply the *law of mass action*, which says that in a chemical reaction,

$$A + B \; \underset{k_2}{\overset{k_1}{\rightleftharpoons}} \; C + D,$$

the rate of forward reaction is proportional to the concentrations of unreacted reactants: $V_{forward} = k_1[A][B]$; also the rate of reverse reaction is proportional to the concentration of the products: $V_{rev} = k_2[C][D]$. At equilibrium, $V_{forward} = V_{rev}$, so that $k_1[A][B] = k_2[C][D]$. Thus the ratio of the rate constants, denoted by $K$, is

$$K = \frac{k_2}{k_1} = \frac{[A][B]}{[C][D]}. \tag{3.1}$$

## Formation of the Drug–Receptor Complex

If A denotes the drug, and R its receptor, the combination of the drug with the receptor is expressed by the reaction

$$A + R \; \underset{k_2}{\overset{k_1}{\rightleftharpoons}} \; AR$$

where AR is the drug–receptor complex, and $k_1$ and $k_2$ are the rate constants of association and dissociation of the complex. If we denote by $X$ the number of AR molecules at any time $t$, by $r_t$ the total number of receptors, and by $A$ the total number of drug molecules,* then the rate of association of complex follows from the mass action law:

$$V_{assoc} = k_1(A - X)(r_t - X).$$

The rate of dissociation is proportional to the amount of complex:

$$V_{dissoc} = k_2 X.$$

The net rate of formation is $dX/dt$, the difference in rates:

$$\frac{dX}{dt} = k_1(A - X)(r_t - X) - k_2 X. \tag{3.2}$$

At equilibrium, the rates of association and dissociation are equal. Hence, $dX/dt = 0$ and from Equation (3.2):

$$k_1(A - X_e)(r_t - X_e) = k_2 X_e. \tag{3.3}$$

---

* We prefer to use number of molecules instead of concentration. For a constant volume of distribution these are proportional.

The subscript e in Equation (3.3) denotes *equilibrium* conditions for $X$. Since $X$ is small compared to $A$, the amount of free drug, $(A - X)$, is approximately equal to $A$. Thus Equation (3.3) becomes

$$k_1 A(r_t - X_e) = k_2 X_e,$$

or

$$X_e = \frac{A r_t}{A + K} \tag{3.4}$$

where $K = k_2/k_1$, the *dissociation constant* of the complex. The graph of Equation (3.4) is shown in Figure 3.1.

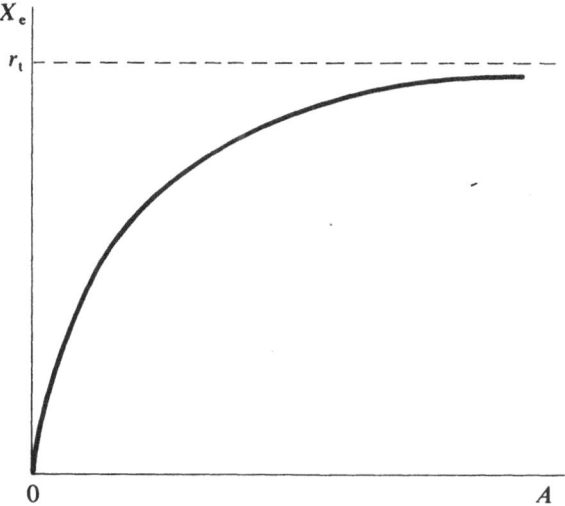

**Figure 3.1** Graph of Equation (3.4).

Numbers of molecules may be converted to concentrations by division by the volume; hence, the practical units of $X_e$, $A$, $r_t$, and $K$ are those of *concentration*. The graph (Fig. 3.1) is strikingly similar to the dose–effect graphs of many drug–effector systems (see Chap. 1). This similarity suggests a simple relationship between $X_e$ and effect. As already pointed out, however, the effect may be very far removed from the AR complex. Even if the effect is intimate, the mathematical relation between $X_e$ and $E$ is generally *unknown* because we do not know what the receptor is and, therefore, cannot measure $X_e$ or $r_t$. Furthermore, the concentration of drug administered need not be the same as the concentration in the vicinity of the receptor, the so-called biophase.

For conditions short of equilibrium, the concentration of complex is obtained by solving Equation (3.2) for $X$. Since $A \gg X$, $A - X \doteq A$, and Equation (3.2) becomes

$$\frac{dX}{dt} = k_1 A(r_t - X) - k_2 X.$$

Solving for $X$ we get

$$X = \frac{Ar_t}{A + K} \{1 - \exp[-(k_1 A + k_2)t]\}.$$

Thus, $X$ rises exponentially to the plateau $Ar_t/(A + K)$, with time constant $(k_1 A + k_2)^{-1}$. The rate of association, $V_{assoc}$, is $k_1 A (r_t - X)$ or, expressing $X$ in terms of $t$,

$$V_{assoc} = k_1 A \left( r_t - \frac{Ar_t}{A + K} \{1 - \exp[-(k_1 A + k_2)t]\} \right)$$

$$= \frac{Ar_t}{A + K} \{k_2 + k_1 A \exp[-(k_1 A + k_2)t]\}.$$

It is seen that $V_{assoc}$ is largest at $t = 0$ and "fades" to the steady value $Ar_t k_2/(A + K)$. The significance of this result will be discussed under Rate Theory.

## Classical Theory

The oldest general theory that related the biological effect $E$ to the concentration $X$ of drug-receptor complex is that of A. J. Clark.[9] The theory as formulated by Clark was extended and made mathematically more rigorous by Ariëns.[1,2] There have been other modifications as we will see subsequently. The Clark–Ariëns view, however, is a useful starting point in our discussion of theories of drug action and may appropriately be called "classical theory."

There are two major assumptions in this theory. First, the magnitude of the effect is *directly proportional* to the concentration $X$ of complex:

$$E = \alpha X. \tag{3.5}$$

Second, the maximal effect occurs when *all* receptors are occupied, i.e., when $X = r_t$. Hence,

$$E_{max} = \alpha r_t. \tag{3.6}$$

When Equations (3.5) and (3.6) are combined with Equation (3.4), the following relation between effect and drug concentration results:

$$E = \frac{\alpha r_t A}{A + K} = \frac{E_{max} A}{A + K}. \tag{3.7}$$

In Equation (3.7), $E$ is the magnitude of the equilibrium effect produced by concentration $A$; $E_{max}$ is the maximum effect. The constant $K$ is the dissociation constant of the drug–receptor complex (more properly, $K$ is the *apparent* dissociation constant, since the real concentration at the receptor is unknown). The reciprocal of $K$ is a measure of the *affinity* of the drug for the receptor.

Equation (3.7) graphs as a hyperbola in rectangular coordinates; thus it has the shape of many actual dose–effect curves, as mentioned earlier. For this reason, Equation (3.7) had been accepted by many pharmacologists as generally applicable. An alternate way of plotting Equation (3.7) is to use the *Hill plot* in which $\log[E/(E_{max} - E)]$ is plotted against $\log A$. By rearrangement of Equation (3.7) we get $E/(E_{max} - E) = A/K$, so that

$$\log\left(\frac{E}{E_{max} - E}\right) = \log A - \log K. \tag{3.8}$$

Thus, the Hill plot is *linear* with slope $= 1$.

The constant of proportionality, $\alpha$, in Equation (3.5) has been termed the *intrinsic activity* by E. J. Ariëns[1,2]; it represents the magnitude of the effect per amount of complex. With the introduction of the concept of intrinsic activity, Ariëns introduced a second constant $\alpha$ in the characterization of drug–receptor interactions; the first was $K$. For a drug to exert an effect on a tissue, it must have both affinity for the receptor and intrinsic activity, or the ability to interact in an "*effective*" way.

Arguments against the assumptions that lead to Equation (3.7) have resulted in several modifications of the classical theory. Among the major objections to this theory is that the assumption of linearity between $E$ and $AR$ is too simple, especially for effects which are composites of other effects (see Chap. 1). Also, several investigators have conducted experiments in which it was proved that a maximum effect could be achieved with something less than full receptor occupancy,[32,36] leading to the idea of *spare receptors*. Several of these modifications of the classical theory are presented in the later sections of this chapter. In spite of the objections, a great deal of drug action is discussed within the framework of the classical theory of Clark and Ariëns. For example, the $E_{max}$ of a drug was called "efficacy" in Chapter 1. According to the classical equation [Equation (3.5)], $E_{max} = \alpha r_t$ so that $\alpha$ is proportional to efficacy when comparing drugs that act on the same receptors. It is common, therefore, to see the terms "efficacy" and "intrinsic activity" used synonymously, an indication that this theory still survives. There are probably several reasons for its survival. Among these is the observation that the theory holds reasonably well for *some* drug–effect combinations. Further, the formulation by A. J. Clark of the theory represented the first important attempt to develop the receptor concept quantitatively, thus providing a framework for interpreting dose–effect data, and forming a basis for Gaddum,[18,19] who later formulated a theory of competitive drug antagonism.

Clark's view that a simple proportionality exists between effect and complex was not explicitly stated as a general rule. Instead it was implied, and there is reason to believe from Clark's own writing that he doubted its general applicability. Clark said, "it seems fair to assume as a general principle that if a pharmacological reaction appears simpler than an analogous reaction in non-living systems, the simplicity must be apparent rather than real."[9] Ariëns[2] is more explicit in qualifying the use of the direct proportion, saying it is "the simplest although not the most probable case." Another reason that classical theory is important is that its kinetics are virtually identical with the kinetics governing enzyme–substrate interaction. Thus, in those situations where receptor is an enzyme, and the effect is the velocity of reaction, the theory can be applied.

If one accepts the assumption leading to Equation (3.7), then this relation permits a determination of $K$ from dose–response data. Substitution of $E = E_{max}/2$ in Equation (3.7) and solving for $A$ yields $A = K$. Thus, $K$ is numerically equal to $A_{50}$, the concentration that produces a half-maximal effect.

The procedure for determining $K$ is as follows:

1. Plot the values of effect versus concentration in rectangular coordinates, using either a linear or logarithmic scale for concentrations.
2. Construct a smooth curve through the plotted points, or a curve that clearly represents the trend, even if it does not contain all the plotted points.
3. From that curve, determine the concentration that produces an effect equal to one-half the maximum. This concentration is numerically equal to $K$ (Fig. 3.2).

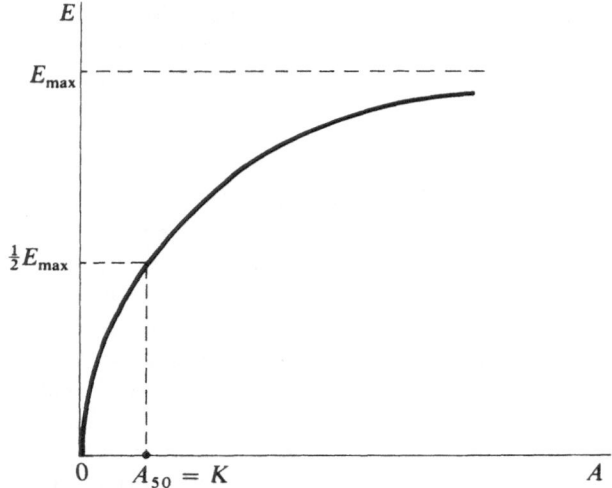

**Figure 3.2** According to "classical" theory the drug–receptor dissociation constant is numerically equal to the concentration that produces a half-maximal effect.

The determination of $K$ by this method has some practical drawbacks in addition to the theoretical assumptions that produced Equation (3.7). One such drawback is that the actual data points may not produce a smooth curve, or it may not be easy to fit the appropriate curve to the points. Another difficulty is that one does not always carry out the experiment to the doses needed to produce $E_{max}$. In such cases a mathematical transformation of Equation (3.7)

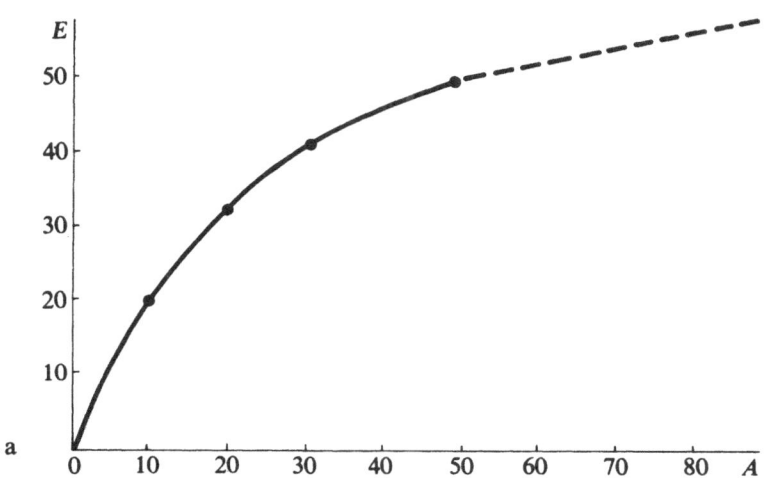

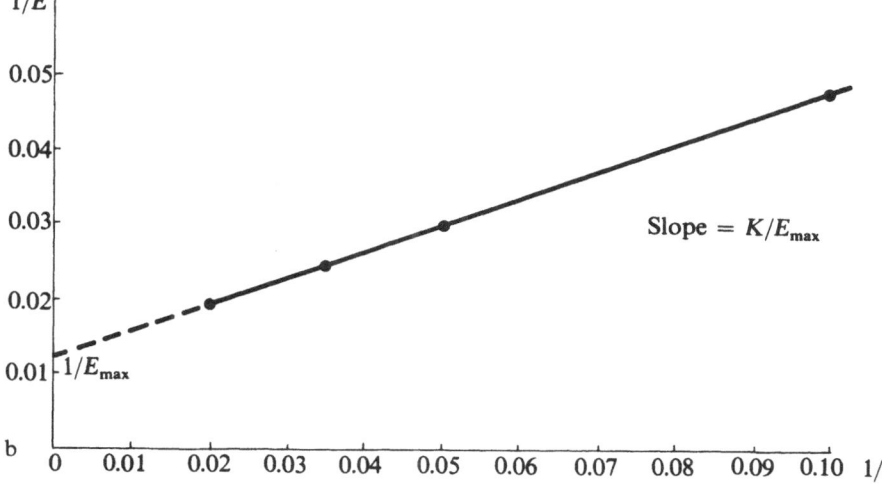

**Figure 3.3** (a) Values of $A$ and $E$ graphed as a hyperbola according to Equation (3.7). (b) Reciprocals of $A$ and $E$ graphed as a straight line. (Theoretical concentration–effect data; arbitrary units.)

may be used. A commonly used transformation is the *double-reciprocal plot*, that is, one plots $1/E$ versus $1/A$ using linear scales. This plot produces, theoretically, a straight line, for when both sides of Equation (3.7) are inverted $1/E = (A + K)/AE_{max}$ or

$$\frac{1}{E} = \frac{K}{E_{max}} \cdot \frac{1}{A} + \frac{1}{E_{max}}. \qquad (3.9)$$

Equation (3.9) is in *linear form* (see Chap. 2). Its slope $= K/E_{max}$; its intercept $= 1/E_{max}$. The graph is illustrated in Figure 3.3. A straight line is then fitted to the reciprocated data. The value of $K$ is the product $(E_{max}) \cdot$ (slope).

An obvious advantage of the double-reciprocal plot is that it is easier to fit a straight line to the measured data than to fit the appropriate hyperbolic curve to the data. Another advantage is that, if $E_{max}$ is not determined experimentally, it may be obtained by extending the line to its intersection with the vertical axis. Such plots are very common in the kinetics of enzymes and substrates and are generally referred to as Lineweaver–Burk plots. It is important to note that the double-reciprocal plot is merely a transformation of Equation (3.7) and *is valid in the analysis of dose–response data only under the assumptions of classical theory*.

Values of $E$ and $A$ are given in the table below and graphed in Figure 3.3a. From these values the reciprocals of $E$ and $A$ are calculated and graphed as in Figure 3.3b. The intercept of the double-reciprocal plot, obtained by extrapolation, is 0.012, from which $E_{max} = 83$.

| $A$ | $E$ | $1/A$ | $1/E$ |
|-----|-----|-------|-------|
| 10 | 21 | 0.10 | 0.048 |
| 20 | 33 | 0.050 | 0.030 |
| 30 | 41 | 0.033 | 0.024 |
| 50 | 50 | 0.020 | 0.020 |

The slope is 0.36. Hence, $K$ is $0.36 \times 83 = 30$ (2 significant figures). Note that the largest measured effect is 50, a value much less than the theoretical maximum of 83.

## Modification of Classical Theory

In an important paper R. P. Stephenson,[36] of the University of Edinburgh, modified the classical theory by the formulation of three postulates:

1. A maximum effect can be produced by an agonist drug *without* total receptor occupancy.
2. The magnitude of the effect is some *unknown function* of the number of receptors occupied. This function is *not* the simple direct proportion, $E =$

$\alpha AR$, of classical theory. (Stephenson does, however, retain the concept that the effect depends on AR, thus preserving the occupation model.)

3. A drug–receptor complex provides a *stimulus S* to the tissue and this stimulus is directly proportional to the fraction of receptors occupied: $S = \varepsilon Y$. In this relation, $Y$ is the fraction of receptors occupied, and $\varepsilon$ is termed *efficacy*. The effect is an unknown function $f$ of the stimulus: $E = f(S)$.

From postulates 2 and 3 we have, therefore, $E = f(S)$ and $S = \varepsilon Y$, where $Y$ is still determined from the mass action law [Equation (3.4)],

$$Y = \frac{X_e}{r_t} = \frac{A}{A + K}.$$

Thus, the function connecting $E$ with $A$ is dissected into a linear, drug-dependent part, $S = \varepsilon Y$, and an unknown, probably nonlinear, drug-independent part, $E = f(S)$. This is an example of a *composite* function.* A consequence of this theory is that *one cannot determine the dissociation constant $K$ (or its reciprocal, the affinity) directly from the dose–response curve as the value $A_{50}$.* Instead, more elaborate experimentation is required to determine $K$ for an agonist. Further mathematical discussion of Stephenson's theory is discussed below.

In addition to rejecting the linearity between effect and occupancy, there are several other conceptual points that represent significant departures from classical theory. Postulate 1 above states that a maximal response can occur even with low receptor occupancy, leading to the concept of *spare receptors*. Drugs that produce a maximal tissue response with appreciable spare receptor capacity have come to be known as *strong agonists* or *full agonists*. It follows from the stimulus relation $S = \varepsilon Y$ that $\varepsilon$, the efficacy, is very large for a strong agonist since $Y$ is small. This concept of efficacy resembles the *intrinsic activity* of Ariëns. It differs, however, in that intrinsic activity relates *effect* to receptor occupancy, whereas efficacy relates stimulus to receptor occupancy. Thus, drugs of different efficacy produce different stimuli, but the relation between stimulus and effect is a property of the tissue and not the drug—a drug-independent property (see also Fig. 1.14).

A drug of low efficacy may produce a response that is less than the tissue maximum even when it is occupying all, or nearly all, of the receptors. Such drugs are called *partial agonists*. Such drugs occupy the same receptor as that of the full agonist and, because they are in competition for the same receptor, diminish the effect of a full agonist when added simultaneously. Partial agonists are, therefore, agents that possess properties intermediate between agonists and pure antagonists. It is noteworthy that postulate 1 says that a maximum effect can be produced by an agonist with less than total receptor occupancy. This statement does not outrule the possibility that *some agonists may produce maximal responses that require full receptor occupancy.* Such drugs would not

---

* See "Chain Rule" in Appendix C, p. 191.

clearly fit into Stephenson's definition of a partial agonist and, therefore, these must be regarded as borderline cases. It is convenient for classification to call such drugs partial agonist also.

We have used the symbol $A_{50}$ to denote the concentration that produces a half-maximal response. With the introduction of partial agonists it is necessary to distinguish between the $E_{max}$ for a particular drug and the $E_{max}$ for the tissue. The term $A_{50}$ for drug A will refer to that concentration which produces a response equal to one half the tissue maximum.

In this theory the relation $E = f(s)$ between effect and stimulus is a property of the system, regardless of the source of the stimulus. Drugs differ in their ability to produce the stimulus. The only thing we know about the function $f$ is that when $S = 0$, $E = 0$. The unit stimulus could be anything; however, *Stephenson adopted the unit for the stimulus to be that which produces a response equal to one half the tissue* $E_{max}$, i.e., $E = E_{max}/2$ when $S = 1$. Since $S = \varepsilon Y$ it follows that for drug A with efficacy $\varepsilon_A$ and dissociation constant $K_A$

$$S = \frac{\varepsilon_A A}{A + k_A}. \tag{3.10}$$

From the definition of the unit for stimulus, Equation (3.10) gives $1 = \varepsilon_A A_{50}/(A_{50} + K_A)$; thus

$$\varepsilon_A = \frac{A_{50} + K_A}{A_{50}} \tag{3.11}$$

The value of $A_{50}$ is determined directly from the dose–response relation for the drug. $K_A$ may be calculated by methods to be described in the following sections of this chapter. Thus, the efficacy $\varepsilon_A$ can be determined from Equation (3.11). Knowing both $\varepsilon_A$ and $K_A$, we can construct the curve for stimulus versus concentration using Equation (3.10). In the case of a strong agonist in which $A_{50} \ll K_A$, Equation (3.11) yields

$$\varepsilon_A \doteq \frac{K_A}{A_{50}}. \tag{3.12}$$

Applications of this theory are given in the several examples below.

In an experiment on isolated thoracic aorta of the rabbit, measurements were made of the developed force in response to graded doses of norepinephrine under conditions of constant length (isometric contraction).[42] In one set of experiments, the muscle was appreciably stretched prior to drug administration. In another set of experiments, the muscle was only lightly stretched before dosing. The dose–response curves are shown in Figure 3.4. The values of $A_{50}$, determined directly from the curves, were $0.18 \times 10^{-7}$ M for condition I (small stretch) and $0.052 \times 10^{-7}$ M for condition II (large stretch). The values of $K$ were also determined, by a method which will be described on p. 67. The $K$ values were found to be $0.84 \times 10^{-7}$ M for condition I and $0.24 \times 10^{-7}$ M for condition II. From Equation (3.11) the efficacy could be calculated: $\varepsilon_A = 5.7$ (condition I) and $\varepsilon_A = 5.6$

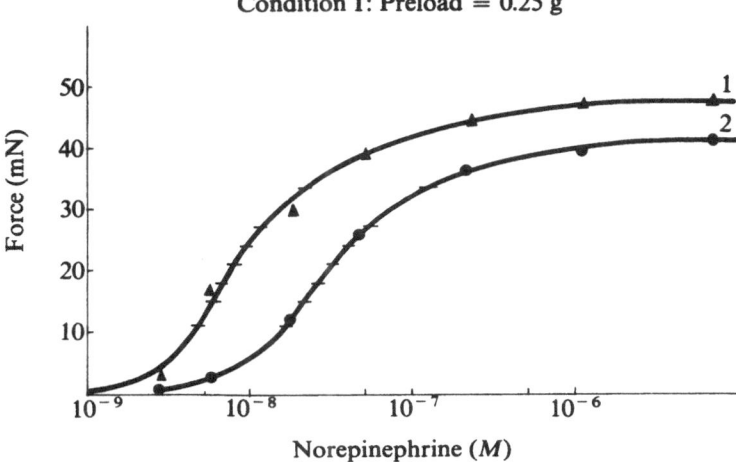

Condition I: Preload = 0.25 g

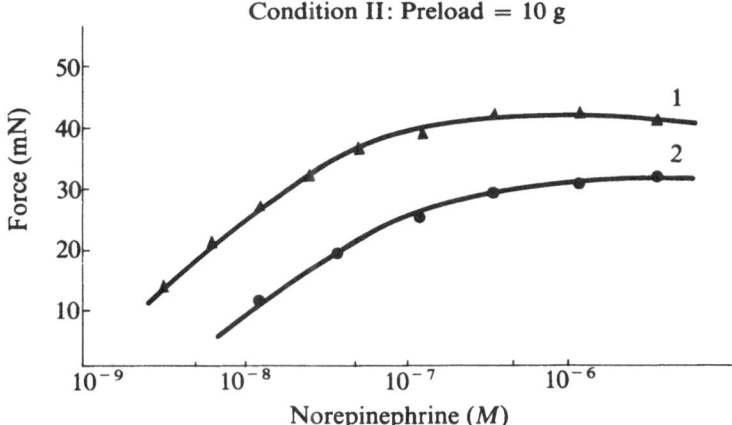

Condition II: Preload = 10 g

**Figure 3.4** Effect of preload on the dissociation construct. *Condition I:* Concentration–response curves to norepinephrine alone (curve 1) and norepinephrine after incubation with $5 \times 10^{-9}$ *M* phenoxybenzamine (curve 2). Developed force is measured in millinewtons (mN). Preload mass = 0.25 g. Horizontal lines show where equiactive concentrations were taken. *Condition II:* Concentration–response curves to norepinephrine alone (curve 1) and norepinephrine after incubation with $5 \times 10^{-9}$ *M* phenoxybenzamine (curve 2). Preload mass = 10 g. Developed force is measured in millinewtons. (Reprinted by permission from Arch Int. Pharmacodyn.[42])

(condition II). The agreement in the values of the efficacy is compatible with the Stephenson's concept of the efficacy as a link between a particular drug and the stimulus it produces. Further, this experiment illustrates the separation of the process into drug-dependent and drug-independent parts. Changing the conditions by stretching affected the stimulus–response relation (the drug-independent part), but it did not change the efficacy (the drug-dependent part).

The function $f$ between stimulus and effect may be determined once the efficacy and $K$ are known. In order to make this determination it is necessary to pair values of $S$ and $A$ [using Equation (3.10)] and values of $E$ and $A$ (from experiment). Then, for each $A$, the corresponding $E$ and $S$ values are known. This is illustrated in the tables below for the data of Figure 3.4 from which the pairs $(A, E)$ are obtained for conditions I and II. The values of $S$ are calculated for each case using the appropriate values of $\varepsilon$ and $K$ in the relation of Equation (3.10).

| Condition I $\left(S = \dfrac{5.7\,A}{A + 0.84 \times 10^{-7}}\right)$ | | | Condition II $\left(S = \dfrac{5.6\,A}{A + 0.24 \times 10^{-7}}\right)$ | | |
|---|---|---|---|---|---|
| $A$ | $E$ | $S$ | $A$ | $E$ | $S$ |
| $5 \times 10^{-9}$ | 11 | 0.32 | $5 \times 10^{-9}$ | 17 | 0.97 |
| $10^{-8}$ | 24 | 0.63 | $10^{-8}$ | 22 | 1.6 |
| $5 \times 10^{-8}$ | 38 | 2.1 | $5 \times 10^{-8}$ | 35 | 3.8 |
| $10^{-7}$ | 41 | 3.1 | $10^{-7}$ | 39 | 4.5 |
| $5 \times 10^{-7}$ | 45 | 4.9 | $5 \times 10^{-7}$ | 40 | 5.3 |
| $10^{-6}$ | 47 | 5.3 | $10^{-6}$ | 40 | 5.5 |

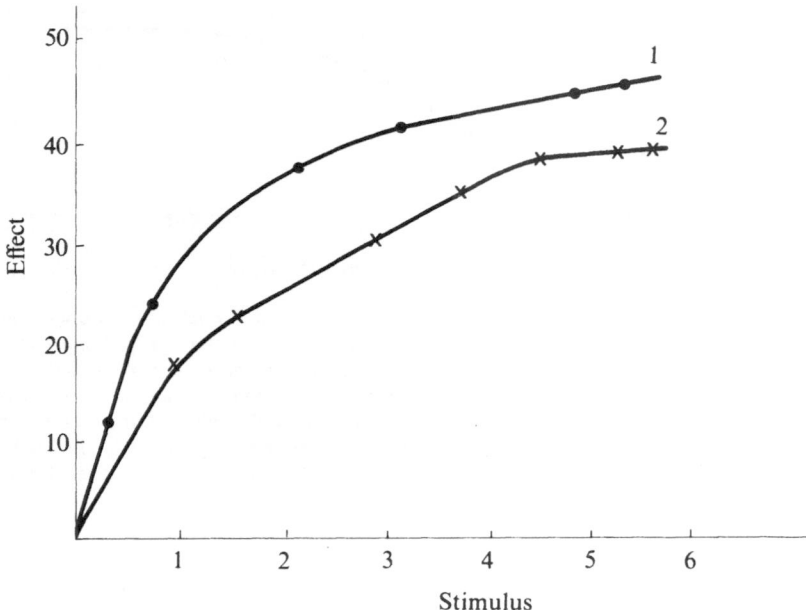

**Figure 3.5** Stimulus–effect relations for isolated rabbit thoracic aorta.

The stimulus–effect functions are shown in Figure 3.5 for each condition. In each case the function is clearly nonlinear. The functions are different because the experimental conditions were different.

Gero[21] recently performed a similar calculation of the stimulus–effect relation from dose–response data for several cholinergic drugs on the fundus of the rabbit stomach. He found a direct proportion between stimulus and effect in this case. The calculation, however, was based on just 3 points from each dose–response curve.

## Dissociation Constants of Competitive Antagonists

The determination of the dissociation constant $K$, of a competitive antagonist, is frequently desirable and, indeed, such determinations provide a quantitative classification of receptors. For example, if an agonist produces two effects, $E_1$ and $E_2$, each thought to be caused by interaction with a single receptor, then the same competitive blocker would be expected to antagonize both effects. This at least identifies the receptors as qualitatively the same. If the values of $K$ for the antagonist, as determined from each effect, are equal, then the receptors are also quantitatively similar.

Another application of the $K$ value of a competitive antagonist is determining whether two agonists act on the same receptor. Two drugs that act on the same receptor should be blocked to the same extent by a competitive antagonist acting at that receptor. If two different $K$'s are obtained for the antagonist, the agonists act on different receptors. If the same value of $K$ is obtained, the evidence strongly suggests a single receptor.

As we have seen (p. 9), the presence of a competitive antagonist is con-centration $B$ produces a displacement to the right of an agonist's dose–response curve. The greater the value of $B$, the greater is the displacement. For a given $B$ one may determine the agonist dose-ratio $A'/A$ for equal effects (see Fig. 1.13) and use the relation

$$\frac{A'}{A} = 1 + \frac{B}{K_B} \tag{3.13}$$

from which $K_B$ may be computed. The derivation of Equation (3.13) is given below. No assumption is made other than the fact that the magnitude of the effect depends on the amount of agonist–receptor complex, without specifying any particular functional relationship.

*Example.* In Figure 3.6, theoretical log dose–response curves are shown and the dose-ratio is obtained at the effect $E_{max}/2$. Since the calibration is logarithmic,

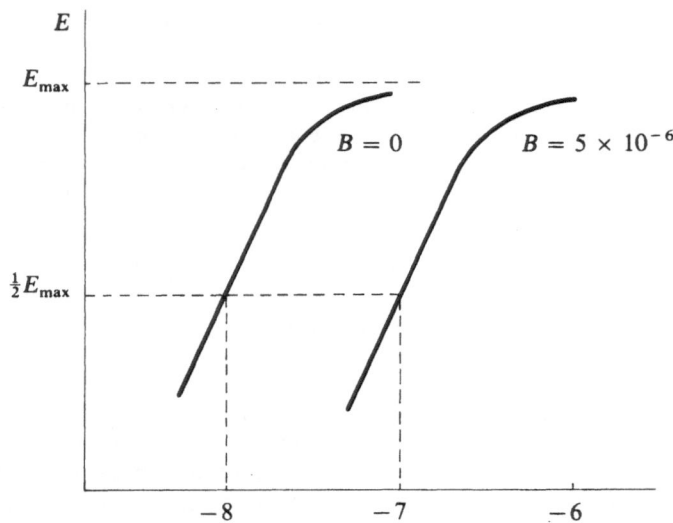

**Figure 3.6** The dose-ratio is $10^{-7}/10^{-8} = 10$, from which $K_B$ is calculated using Equation (3.13).

the doses are $A = 10^{-8}$ $M$ and $A' = 10^{-7}$ $M$, yielding the ratio $A'/A = 10$. If, for example, $B = 5 \times 10^{-6}$ $M$, we get from Equation (3.13) $10 = 1 + 5 \times 10^{-6}/K_B$, from which $K_B = 5.5 \times 10^{-7}$ $M$.

In practice the calculation of $K_B$ is made from not just one, but from several ($n$) concentrations of antagonist. We get the dose-ratio $A'/A$ for each of the $n$ concentrations of $B$, that is, $(A'/A)_i$, and $B_i$, for $i = 1$ to $i = n$. The values of the dose-ratio for each $B_i$ are plotted in terms of logarithms (base 10): $\log(A'/A - 1)$ versus $\log B$. The purpose of this plot may be seen by taking logs of both sides of Equation (3.13). We get $\log(A'/A - 1) = \log B - \log K_B$, an expression in *linear form* (see p. 26).

Thus when $\log(A'/A - 1)$ is plotted against $\log B$, one obtains a straight line of slope *unity* and *intercept* ($-\log K_B$), as in Figure 3.7. This method of plotting, used by Arunlakshana and Schild,[3] is perferred over the single dose-ratio determination since it minimizes the error of a single determination. The plotted points should fit a straight line of slope unity; thus the method also provides a means of checking the applicability of the model.

The negative common logarithm of $K_B$ (in molar units) is called the "$pA_2$"[3,34]:

$$pA_2 = -\log K_B. \tag{3.14}$$

For example, a value of $K_B$ equal to $10^{-7}$ $M$ (which means affinity $= 10^{+7}$) gives $pA_2 = 7$. Values of $pA_2$ are frequently used for competitive antagonists

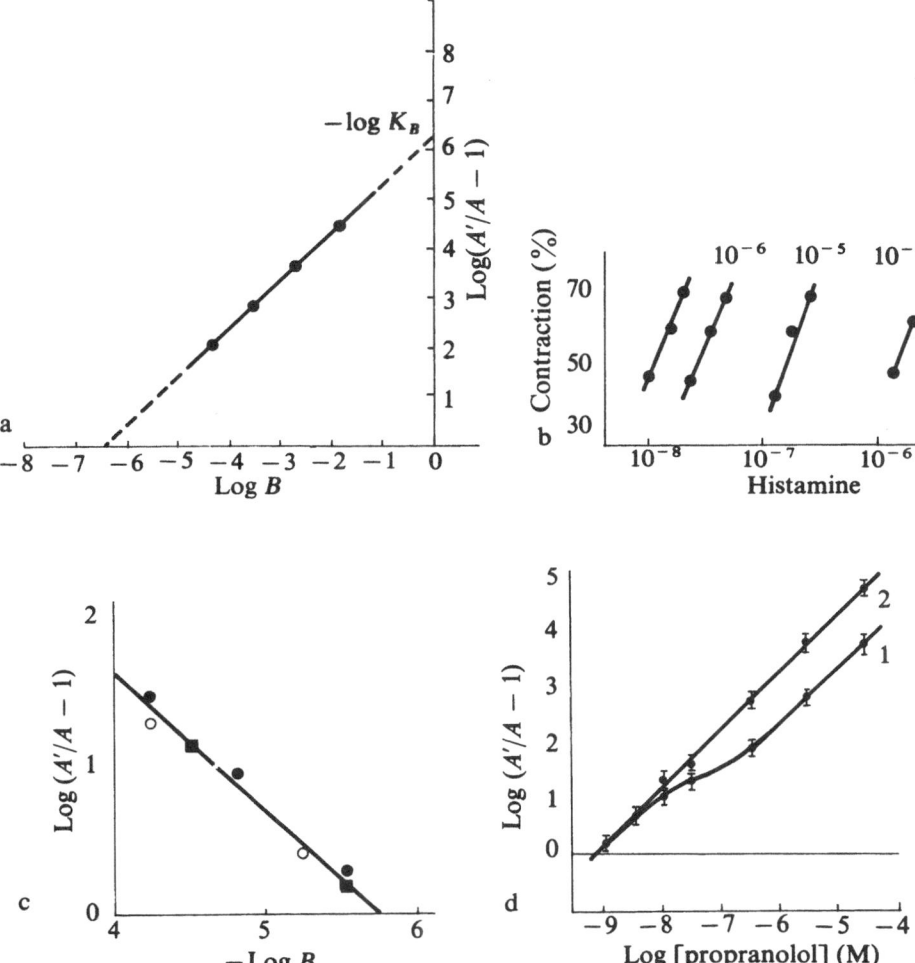

**Figure 3.7** (a) Determination of $K_B$ for a competitive antagonist using several concentrations of the antagonist (theoretical). Since the molar concentrations are negative powers of 10, such as $10^{-6}$, $10^{-5}$, etc., the values of log $B$ are −6, −5, etc. Thus, the plotted values in the graph are in the negative domain. The intercept, in this case 6.2, equals −log $K_B$; hence, $K_B = 10^{-6.2}$. The $pA_2 = 6.2$. (b) Dose−response data showing effect of histamine on guinea pig ileum and the shifts produced by different concentrations of the antagonist atropine (A).[3] (c) Schild plots from experiments of the kind shown in (b).[3] (d) Illustration of the nonlinearity of Schild plots (curve 1) and the effect of blocking the extraneuronal uptake (curve 2) responsible for the nonlinearity.[14] Curves in (b) and (c) redrawn with permission of Br. J. Pharmacol.; curve (d) redrawn with permission of Fed. Proc.

instead of their $K_B$ values. As an example, Furchgott[13] used $pA_2$ values when reporting his studies with the $\beta$-antogonist pronethalol. He measured the $pA_2$ for pronethalol in antogonizing $\beta$-mediated effects in the rabbit aorta and duodenum. The values of $pA_2$ were 7.5 for the aorta and 6.4 for the duodenum. These correspond to $K_B$ values of $10^{-7.5}$ (aortic $\beta$-receptors) and $10^{-6.4}$ (duodenal $\beta$-receptors). It is noteworthy that the difference in $pA_2$ values found in this study was the first bit of quantitative evidence for the existence of two kinds of $\beta$-receptors and, thus, demonstrates the importance of this measure in receptor differentiation. In other words, both $\beta$-receptors are antagonized by pronethalol, but the affinities as determined by the $pA_2$ suggest a quantitative difference.

A graph of the kind illustrated in Figure 3.7 is called a *Schild plot*. Some workers make these plots using $-\log B$ on the abscissa. If this is done the line will have slope $-1$. Figure 3.7 shows dose–response data and the corresponding Schild plots constructed by Arunlakshana and Schild[3] from their data collected from the guinea pig ileum. The dose–response curves, constructed with abscissa calibrated logarithmically, illustrate the parallelism. (See p. 103 for a discussion of methods for fitting parallel lines.)

In constructing Schild plots, some curve fitting procedure, such as the method of least squares (see p. 98), is almost always used. In some cases the slope of the resulting line turns out to be different from unity. In these cases, the common practice is to take the $pA_2$ as the intercept on the abscissa. This practice is somewhat questionable, however, since competitive theory requires unit slope, in which case both intercepts yield the same value. In some cases, the departure from unit slope, and even nonlinearity can be explained, in which case correction may be made, as discussed by Furchgott.[14,17] In other cases, we do not know the reason for departure from unit slope. In these cases we can fit the data to the best line of unit slope using the least squares criterion as discussed in Chapter 4 for this special case. Tallarida and co-workers[38] applied this alternate method in the determination of the $pA_2$ in a situation in which the slope of the Schild plot was slightly different from unity, namely, 1.06. In this case the $pA_2$ and its standard error was $7.95 \pm 0.19$. When the same data were fitted to the best line of unit slope, the corresponding $pA_2$ was $8.01 \pm 0.07$. The difference in $pA_2$ values in this case was rather small. However, in cases in which the slope of the standard plot differs appreciably from unity, the two methods of plotting give rather different values for the $pA_2$ and its standard error. (See Table 5.1 for a list of $pA_2$ values and the slopes of the corresponding Schild plots.)

The example mentioned above used data from an intact animal (rat). The special problems arising with such in vivo $pA_2$ values are discussed in Chapter 5. However, departures from unit slope, and even nonlinear Schild plots, arise sometimes in studies conducted on isolated preparations. As an illustration, Figure 3.7d is a Schild plot obtained by Furchgott and co-workers for propranolol–isoproterenol in isolated strips of guinea pig trachea in which the response was relaxation of the smooth muscle.[14,17] The nonlinear plot was explained by Furchgott as being due to an active uptake of isoproterenol by the extraneural uptake mechanism, and is accounted for in equations that he derived. When this uptake was blocked by pretreatment with dibenamine, the data gave the theoretically predicted linear plot (curve 2) with a slope of 1.006. Kenakin and Black[27] reported a similar phenomenon in their study of iso-prenaline–practolol interaction in rat atria.

A further discussion of the statistical procedures used in the determination of the $pA_2$ is given on pages 101 and 103; the special problems encountered in vivo are discussed in Chapter 5. The literature contains a number of articles which discuss methods, mathematical and pharmacological, for determining the $pA_2$. See, for example, the articles by Waud,[46] MacKay,[29] Stone and Angus,[37] and Tallarida et al.[38]

### The Competitive Equation

In competitive antagonism the agonist, A, and the antagonist, B, react reversibly with a common receptor R:

$$A + R \underset{k_{2A}}{\overset{k_{1A}}{\rightleftarrows}} AR$$

$$B + R \underset{k_{2B}}{\overset{k_{1B}}{\rightleftarrows}} BR$$

The total receptor population will be denoted by $r_t$. At any time $t$ let the number of AR complexes be given by $X$, and BR complexes by $Y$. These combinations reduce the unoccupied receptor population to $(r_t - X - Y)$. The available agonist is, therefore, $A - X$; also the available antagonist is $B - Y$. As $A \gg X$ and $B \gg Y$, we have $A - X \doteq A$ and $B - Y \doteq B$. Application of the mass action law to these simultaneous reactions yields the equations for rates of formation

$$\frac{dX}{dt} = k_{1A} A(r_t - X - Y) - K_{2A} X \tag{3.15}$$

and

$$\frac{dY}{dt} = k_{1B} B(r_t - X - Y) - k_{2B} Y. \tag{3.16}$$

At equilibrium $dX/dt = dY/dt = 0$, and Equations (3.15) and (3.16) give

$$A(r_t - X - Y) = K_A X \tag{3.17}$$

and

$$B(r_t - X - Y) = K_B Y, \tag{3.18}$$

where $K_A = k_{2A}/k_{1A}$ and $K_B = k_{2B}/k_{1B}$.

From Equation (3.18), we obtain $Y$, the concentration of $BR$ at equilibrium:

$$Y = \frac{B(r_t - X)}{B + K_B}.$$ (3.19)

Substitution of $Y$ from Equation (3.19) into Equation (3.17), and rearranging, we obtain $X$, the equilibrium concentration of $AR$:

$$X = \frac{Ar_t}{A + K_A[1 + (B/K_B)]}.$$ (3.20)

In the absence of the antagonist, $B = 0$, and Equation (3.20) gives the usual equation

$$X = \frac{Ar_t}{A + K_A}.$$ (3.21)

A salient feature of Equation (3.20) is that for any value of $A$, $X$ is less than it would be according to Equation (3.21) in which there is no blocker. Hence, *for equal values of $X$, which means equal responses, the concentration of $A$ in Equation (3.20) would have to be increased to $A'$. Thus*

$$\frac{Ar_t}{A + K_A} = \frac{A'r_t}{A' + K_A[1 + (B/K_B)]}$$

from which it follows that

$$\frac{A'}{A} + 1 = \frac{B}{K_B},$$

which is the dose-ratio equation.

As we said previously there is *no assumption of direct proportionality* between effect $E$ and agonist–receptor complex $X$. If, however, we make the assumptions $E = \alpha X$, and $E_{max} = \alpha r_t$, we obtain $E = E_{max}A/(A + K_A)$ in the unblocked case, and $E = AE_{max}/[A + K_A(1 + B/K_B)]$ in the presence of the competitive antagonist. The double-reciprocal (Lineweaver–Burk)* relations for the two cases are

$$\frac{1}{E} = \frac{1}{E_{max}} + \frac{K_A}{E_{max}} \cdot \frac{1}{A}$$ (3.22)

and

$$\frac{1}{E} = \frac{1}{E_{max}} + \frac{K_A(1 + B/K_B)}{E_{max}} \cdot \frac{1}{A}.$$ (3.23)

* The double-reciprocal plots here are formally equivalent to those discussed in Chapter 2 for enzyme–substrate interactions.

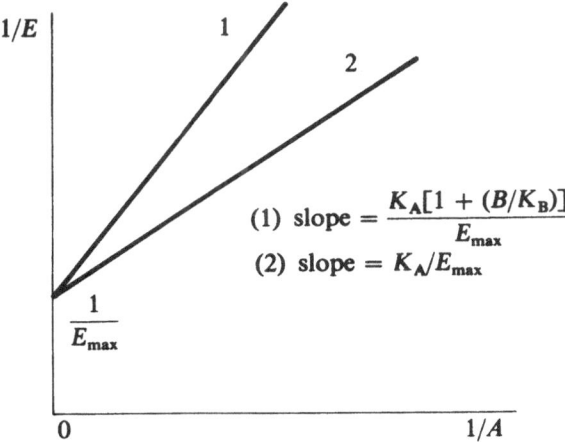

**Figure 3.8** Double-reciprocal plot for a competitive antagonist. According to the classical theory the intercept is the same. In the presence of antagonist the slope is greater by the factor $(1 + B/K_B)$. Curve 1, antagonist and agonist; curve 2, agonist alone.

It is seen that the straight line relations of Equations (3.22) and (3.23) have the same intercept, $1/E_{max}$. The slope from Equation (3.23) is $K_A(1 + B/K_B)/E_{max}$ which is larger by the factor $(1 + B/K_B)$ than the slope of Equation (3.22) (Fig. 3.8). *It should be emphasized that these double-reciprocal plots of effect versus dose yield values for $K_A$ and $K_B$ only if one accepts the assumptions of classical theory.*

## Dissociation Constants of Agonists: Method of Partial Irreversible Blockade

According to classical theory, one may determine the dissociation constant of an agonist directly from the dose–response curve. The value so obtained, however, may not be correct since the assumptions of classical theory are questionable. The method that is generally accepted is that employed by Furchgott and Bursztyn[15] in which the assumptions of the classical theory are not made. The method uses an irreversible antagonist that combines with the same receptor as that of the agonist. Furchgott and Bursztyn studied the effect of muscarinic agonists on isolated stomach muscle of the rabbit, using dibenamine as the antagonist. The only assumption in this method is that the effect depends on the amount of agonist–receptor complex; hence, equal effects, in the presence of or in the absence of the antagonist, mean equal amounts of agonist–receptor complex. The antagonist, by combining irreversibly with the receptor, reduces the free receptor population permanently. Figure 3.9

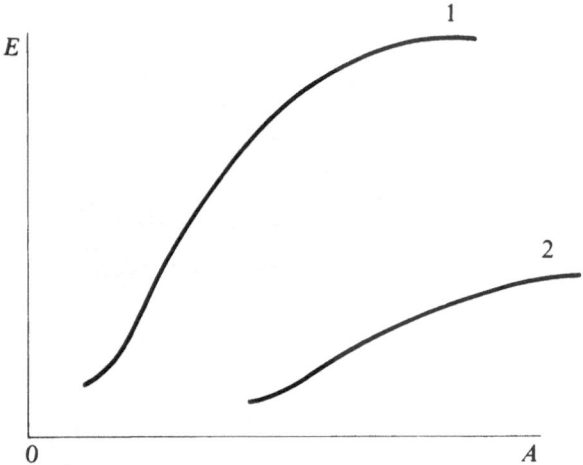

**Figure 3.9** Partial irreversible blockade. Curve 2 represents the dose–response curve for the agonist after pretreatment with the noncompetitive antagonist. Curve 2 does not achieve the same maximum as curve 1, which is the agonist dose–response curve in the unblocked situation.

illustrates the dose–response curves obtained in a typical experiment of this kind. Some number $N$ of equal effects is taken corresponding to agonist concentrations $(A_1, A_1'), (A_2, A_2'), \ldots, (A_N, A_N')$. These pairs of concentrations are plotted as reciprocals, $1/A$ versus $1/A'$, which (theoretically) obey a straight line equation.

$$\frac{1}{A} = \frac{1}{q} \cdot \frac{1}{A'} + \frac{1/q - 1}{K}. \tag{3.24}$$

In this equation, $q$ *is the fraction of receptors that remain.* The slope in Equation (3.24) is $1/q$, and the intercept (on the vertical axis) is $(1/q - 1)/K$. It follows that $K$ may be determined from such a plot as follows:

$$K = \frac{(\text{slope} - 1)}{\text{intercept}}. \tag{3.25}$$

Figure 3.10 is a theoretical plot that illustrates the method. Figure 3.11 shows actual data.

This method has been applied by different investigators in order to determine $K$ for catecholamines on the $\alpha$-adrenergic receptor of isolated strips of rabbit aorta. The values are shown in Table 3.1. The differences in the values reported by different investigators give some idea of the sensitivity of the method to variations in the experimental procedure. The individual references should be consulted for details (see also Chap. 6).

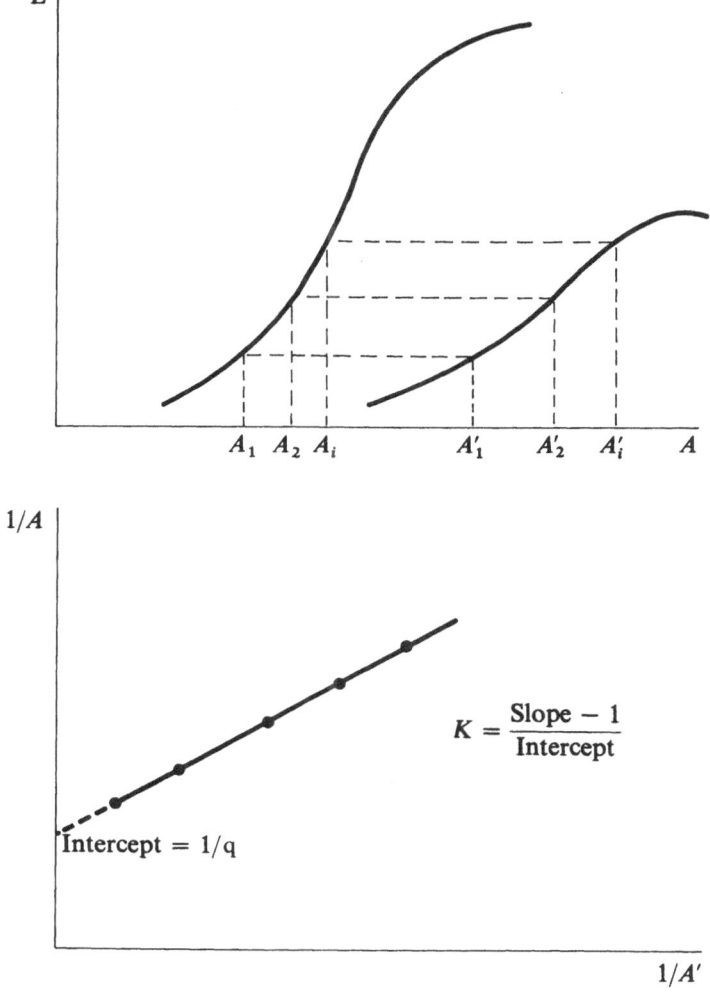

**Figure 3.10** The method of partial irreversible blockade for determining the dissociation constant of an agonist.

Broadly and Nicholson[6] made use of this method to study $\beta$-receptors in guinea pig heart. Using both rate and tension responses, they found no difference between the $K$ values for each.

The method of partial irreversible blockade is the generally accepted method for determining the dissociation constant of an agonist drug. Its application to a particular drug–effector system requires, however, the use of a second agent which can irreversibly inactivate a fraction of the total receptor population. Like the method used for competitive antagonists, this agonist method

**Table 3.1**

Dissociation constants ($\pm$ S.E.M.) in molar units for several catecholamines in rabbit aortic strips

| Investigator | l-Norepinephrine | l-Epinephrine | l-Phenylephrine | Dopamine |
|---|---|---|---|---|
| Besse and Furchgott[5] | $(3.39 \pm 0.15) \times 10^{-7}$ | $(2.07 \pm 0.31) \times 10^{-7}$ | $(1.13 \pm 0.14) \times 10^{-6}$ | $(6.36 \pm 0.42) \times 10^{-5}$ |
| Sheys and Green[35] | $(1.31 \pm 0.54) \times 10^{-7}$ | $(2.94 \pm 0.84) \times 10^{-7}$ | $(1.27 \pm 0.13) \times 10^{-6}$ | $(1.53 \pm 0.66) \times 10^{-5}$ |
| Jacob and Tallarida[23] | $(0.84 \pm 0.16) \times 10^{-7}$ | | | |

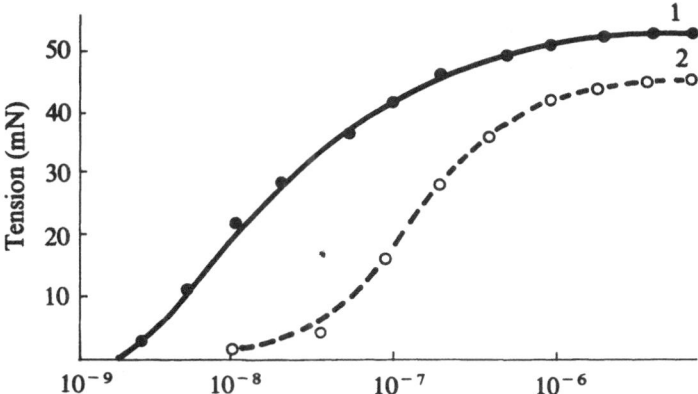

**Figure 3.11** Norepinephrine concentration–response curve obtained on a spirally cut strip of rabbit thoracic aorta in the absence of (curve 1) and in the presence of (curve 2) phenoxybenzamine. Data for curve 2 were obtained after washing to zero baseline followed by incubation with $5 \times 10^{-9}$ $M$ phenoxybenzamine. Responses are recorded as isometric tension. Redrawn from Tallarida et al.[41] with permission of IEEE Transactions Biomed. Engineering.

is based on so-called occupation theory, but, unlike the "classical theory," *it requires no assumption of linearity between the effect and the agonist–receptor complex concentration.* Another method for dealing with agonists of a certain kind is discussed in the next section.

The derivation of Equation (3.24) follows from Equation (3.4) which relates the amount of drug–receptor complex $X$ to the drug concentration $A$ and receptor concentration $r_t$,

$$X = \frac{Ar_t}{A + K}.$$

If a fraction of the receptors is blocked, leaving $qr_t$ ($q < 1$), then the drug concentration must be increased to $A'$ in order to achieve the *same effect. Thus,*

$$\frac{A'qr_t}{A' + K} = \frac{Ar_t}{A + K}.$$

Rearrangement of the above equation yields Equation (3.24). The reciprocated data are fitted to a straight line using an appropriate curve fitting procedure such as the method of least squares (see p. 98).

*Example.* In the study by Tallarida et al.[41] (Fig. 3.11) rabbit aorta was contracted by norepinephrine alone (case 1) and by norepinephrine in the presence of the noncompetitive antagonist phenoxybenzamine (case 2). Matching

**Table 3.2**
Equiactive molar concentrations of
norepinephrine in the absence (case
1) and in the presence (case 2) of a
fixed concentration of blocker

| $A$ (Case 1) | $A'$ (Case 2) |
|---|---|
| $0.20 \times 10^{-7}$ | $1.1 \times 10^{-7}$ |
| $0.14 \times 10^{-7}$ | $0.71 \times 10^{-7}$ |
| $0.12 \times 10^{-7}$ | $0.50 \times 10^{-7}$ |
| $0.091 \times 10^{-7}$ | $0.38 \times 10^{-7}$ |
| $0.076 \times 10^{-7}$ | $0.32 \times 10^{-7}$ |
| $0.067 \times 10^{-7}$ | $0.26 \times 10^{-7}$ |
| $0.055 \times 10^{-7}$ | $0.22 \times 10^{-7}$ |
| $0.048 \times 10^{-7}$ | $0.17 \times 10^{-7}$ |

responses were obtained from concentrations of norepinephrine (Table 3.2). When $1/A$ versus $1/A'$ was plotted the resulting straight line had slope 3.1 and intercept $2.5 \times 10^7$. Thus, from Equation (3.25):

$$K = (3.1 - 1)/(2.5 \times 10^7)$$
$$= 0.84 \times 10^{-7} \, M.$$

## Dissociation Constants of Agonists: Method of Partial Agonists

An alternate method for determining the dissociation constant of agonists has been used by Barlow et al.[4] and by Waud.[4,5] In contrast to the method of the previous section, this method does not make use of irreversible antagonists; it is applicable, however, only to partial agonists. It may be recalled (see p. 57) that a full* agonist has a large spare receptor capacity. A partial agonist, however, requires an appreciable receptor occupancy and may or may not achieve the tissue's maximal response.

In this method, dose–response curves for a partial agonist and a full agonist are obtained. The *concentrations of each which produce equal responses* are determined as in Figure 3.12. These concentrations are denoted $(A_1, P_1)$, $(A_2, P_2), \ldots, (A_n, P_n)$, where $A_i$ is the dose of the full agonist and $P_i$ is the corresponding dose of the partial agonist. A plot of $1/A$ versus $1/P$ will be linear with slope, intercept, and $K_P$ (for the partial agonist) related as follows:

$$K_P = \frac{\text{slope}}{\text{intercept}}. \tag{3.26}$$

---

* Also called a "strong" agonist.

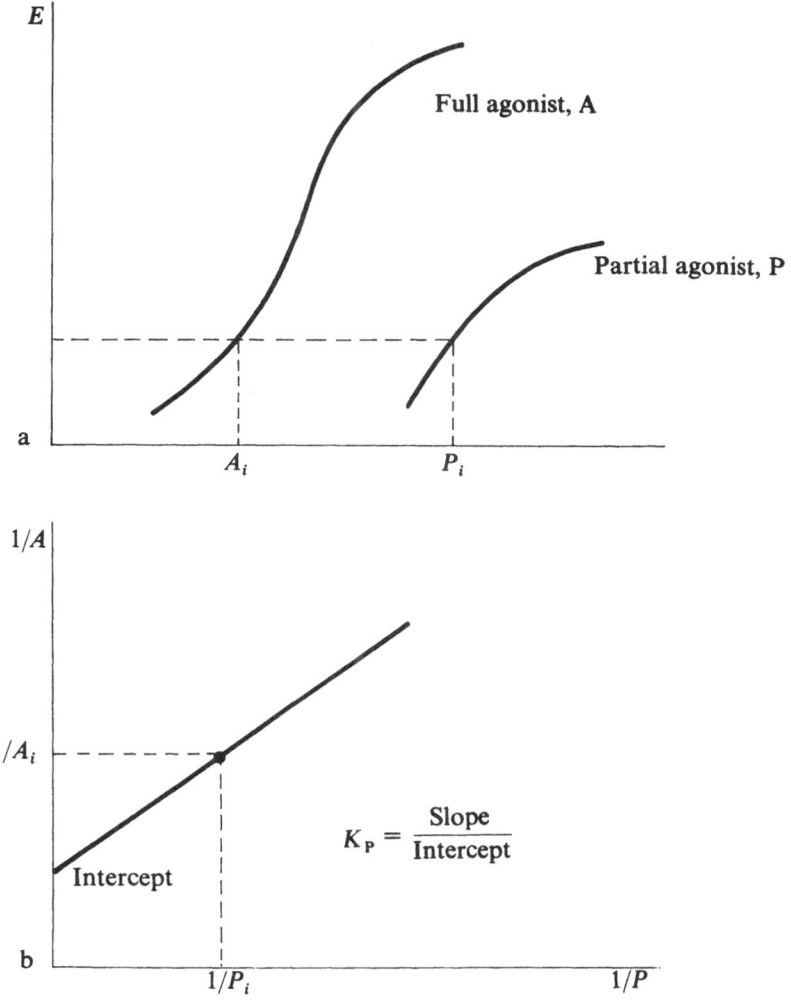

**Figure 3.12** (a) The determination of $K$ for the concentration of a partial agonist, $P$, compares equal responses with the corresponding concentrations of a strong agonist, $A$. (b) The reciprocals of equiactive concentrations from curve (a) are plotted producing a straight line.

When this method was applied to certain muscarinic agents, using carbachol as the full agonist, the values of $K$ agreed well with those obtained by the method of irreversible blockage. The theory underlying this method utilizes Stephenson's[36] modification of classical theory (see p. 56).

In this formulation we start with the equation relating the concentration of complex $X$ to the concentration $D$: $X = (r_t D)/(D + K)$. It is convenient to use fractional occupancy $Y = X/r_t = D/(D + K)$. For a strong agonist, drug A, we have the fraction $Y_A$ of occupied receptors given by the approximate equation

$$Y_A \doteq \frac{A}{K_A}. \tag{3.27}$$

The partial agonist P, however, requires concentrations $P$ sufficiently high that one must use the relation

$$Y_P = \frac{P}{P + K_P}. \tag{3.28}$$

The effect of each is a function of the fractional occupancy

$$E_A = g(e_A Y_A) \quad \text{and} \quad E_P = g(e_P Y_P),$$

where each $e$ represents the "efficacy" in Stephenson's formulation. Equating equal responses, $E_A = E_P$, we get

$$e_A \frac{A}{K_A} = e_P \frac{P}{P + K_P}.$$

Reciprocating,

$$\frac{K_A}{e_A} \cdot \frac{1}{A} = \frac{1}{e_P} + \frac{K_P}{e_P} \cdot \frac{1}{P}$$

or

$$\frac{1}{A} = \frac{e_A}{e_P K_A} + \frac{e_A}{K_A} \cdot \frac{K_P}{e_P} \cdot \frac{1}{P}.$$

The plot of $1/A$ versus $1/P$ is, therefore, a straight line with slope $= e_A/e_P \cdot K_P/K_A$ and intercept $= e_A/e_P K_A$. Hence, slope/intercept $= K_P$, which is Equation (3.26).

*Example.* Table 3.3 gives equiactive concentrations of a strong agonist butyl-TMA and a partial agonist nonyl-TMA in producing contraction of the guinea pig ileum. A plot of $1/A$ against $1/P$ produced a line with slope 13 and intercept $0.046 \times 10^7$. From Equation (3.26) we get $K = 2.8 \times 10^{-5}$.

**Table 3.3**
Equiactive concentrations of a strong agonist (A) and a partial agonist (P)[a]

| A (butyl-TMA) | P (nonyl-TMA) |
| --- | --- |
| $3.0 \times 10^{-7}$ | $4.5 \times 10^{-6}$ |
| $4.0 \times 10^{-7}$ | $6.6 \times 10^{-6}$ |
| $5.0 \times 10^{-7}$ | $8.0 \times 10^{-6}$ |
| $8.0 \times 10^{-7}$ | $14.0 \times 10^{-6}$ |
| $10.0 \times 10^{-7}$ | $50.0 \times 10^{-6}$ |

[a] Data from Stephenson.[36]

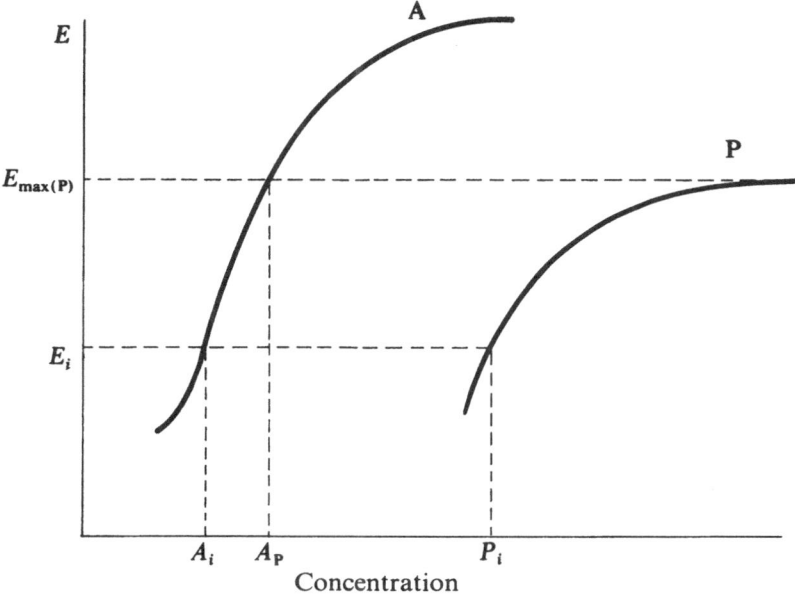

**Figure 3.13** Matching the responses of a full agonist (A) and a partial agonist (P).

This method of determining $K$ for a partial agonist requires that the full agonist have the property $K_A \gg A$. If the full agonist does not have this property the method will not work. Gero and Tallarida[22] considered this case and developed an alternate method for the determination of $K_P$ for the partial agonist P. This method also involves matching the responses of P with those of a full agonist A. With reference to Figure 3.13, let us denote by $A_P$ that concentration of A which produces a tissue response equal to the maximum of drug P. Also, we select any other pair of concentrations $P_i$ and $A_i$ which yield the same effect $E_i$. With *no assumptions regarding the relative values of* $K_A$, $A_P$, and $A_i$, it can be shown that $K_P$ and $K_A$ are related as

$$K_P = \frac{K_A(A_P - A_i) \cdot P_i}{(A_P + K_A) \cdot A_i}.$$  (3.29)

(See derivation below.) Hence, if $K_A$ is known for the full agonist, $K_P$ may be calculated from Equation (3.29).

Since the maximum effect of $P$ is achieved with full receptor occupancy it follows (from the formula $S = \varepsilon Y$) that the maximum stimulus produced by P is $\varepsilon_P$, its efficacy. This same value of stimulus is achieved by drug A with something less than full receptor occupancy and with concentration $A_P$. Thus for drug A we have $S_A = \varepsilon_A A_P/(A_P + K_A)$. Equating $\varepsilon_P$ to $S_A$ gives $\varepsilon_P = \varepsilon_A A_P/(A_P + K_A)$ or

$$\frac{\varepsilon_A}{\varepsilon_P} = 1 + \frac{K_A}{A_P}.$$  (3.30)

For any other level of effect $E_i$ produced by A and P their stimuli must be the same, or

$$\frac{\varepsilon_A A_i}{A_i + K_A} = \frac{\varepsilon_P P_i}{P_i + K_P}$$

from which

$$\frac{\varepsilon_A}{\varepsilon_P} = \frac{P_i}{P_i + K_P} \cdot \frac{A_i + K_A}{A_i}. \tag{3.31}$$

Equating the right-hand sides of Equations (3.30) and (3.31) gives

$$1 + \frac{K_A}{A_P} = \frac{P_i}{P_i + K_P} \cdot \frac{A_i + K_A}{A_i}$$

and solving for $K_P$

$$K_P = \frac{K_A(A_P - A_i)P_i}{A_i(A_P + K_A)}$$

which is Equation (3.29).

*Example.* In an experiment with full and partial adrenergic agonists the following (molar) values were obtained: $A_i = 10^{-9}$; $A_P = 5 \times 10^{-9}$; $P_i = 10^{-7}$. The full agonist was known to have the value $K_A = 5 \times 10^{-8}$ (determined by the method on p. 68). The value of $K_P$ is, from Equation (3.29),

$$K_P = \frac{5 \times 10^{-8}(5 \times 10^{-9} - 10^{-9})10^{-7}}{10^{-9}(5 \times 10^{-9} + 5 \times 10^{-8})}$$

$$= 3.6 \times 10^{-7} \, M.$$

## Perturbation Methods

We have seen that the method generally accepted for determining the dissociation constant for a strong agonist drug with its receptor involves the use of an irreversible antagonist that reacts with the same receptor. If the drug is a partial agonist, then one can determine its $K$ value by matching equal effects with those produced by a strong agonist that combines with the same receptor. In each of these methods, therefore, a second drug is needed. Only if one accepts the assumption of a direct proportion between effect and concentration is it possible to determine $K$ directly from the dose–response data. Hence, the problem of determining $K$ depends upon the availability of a second drug, or it involves a rather questionable theoretical assumption. It is not surprising, therefore that researchers have sought other methods which might be applicable to this determination, even if such methods have limited application. One such method is a perturbation or "relaxation" method. In this method the equilibrium is perturbed and the kinetics of the restoration process are observed from which, not only $K$, but also the forward and reverse rate constants $k_1$ and $k_2$ may be determined.

For a given concentration $A$ of agonist the concentration of drug–receptor complex at equilibrium will be some value $X_e$. If the equilibrium is disturbed by means of some small perturbation, the concentration of complex changes from $X = X_e$ to $X = X_e + \mu$. It may be shown[40] that the magnitude of the change, denoted by $\mu$, attains a maximum value $\mu_{max}$, and recovers in time according to

$$\mu = \mu_{max}[\exp\{-(k_1 A + k_2)t\}]. \tag{3.32}$$

The effect will change from its equilibrium value $E$ to $E + \Delta E$ and, for sufficiently small $\mu$, it follows that the change in response obeys the equation

$$\Delta E = \Delta E_{max}[\exp\{-(k_1 A + k_2 t)\}]. \tag{3.33}$$

In Equation (3.33) $\Delta E_{max}$ is the maximum change in response. It is convenient to define the time constant for recovery $\tau$:

$$\tau = (k_1 A + k_2)^{-1}, \tag{3.34}$$

from which Equation (3.33) becomes

$$\Delta E = \Delta E_{max} \exp(-t/\tau). \tag{3.35}$$

From Equation (3.35) it follows that when $t = \tau$, $\Delta E = \Delta E_{max} \cdot \exp(-1) = 0.37\,\Delta E_{max}$. Thus, the *time constant is that time necessary for $\Delta E$ to change from $\Delta E_{max}$ to $(0.37)\Delta E_{max}$, as shown in Figure 3.14.*

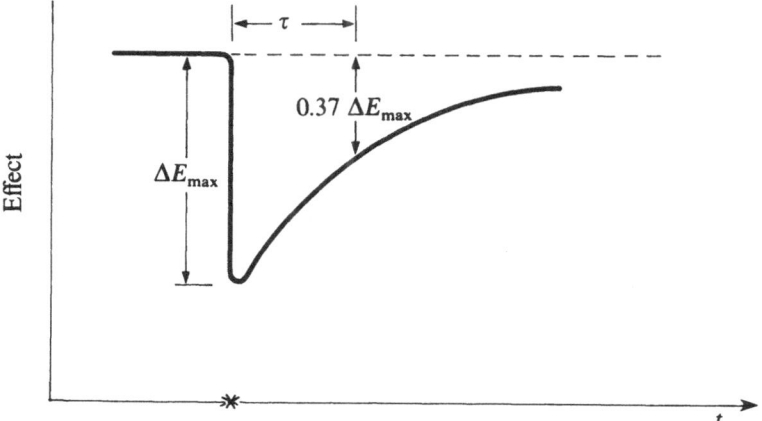

**Figure 3.14** Perturbation method for determining rate constants of the drug–receptor reaction. The time constant is the time required for the system to recover to $(0.37)\Delta E_{max}$.

With reference to Figure 3.14, a perturbation is introduced at the instant marked with * producing a rapid change in response which reaches a maximum, $\Delta E_{max}$. The time constant $\tau$ is determined from the recovery record as shown in the figure. The value of $\tau$ is related to the concentration $A$ according to Equation (3.34). If perturbations are made at two different concentrations, $A_1$ and $A_2$, and the respective time constants for recovery, $\tau_1$ and $\tau_2$, are determined, the values may be used in Equation (3.34) to yield two equations from which $k_1$ and $k_2$ may be determined. A more precise method is to perturb at several values of drug concentration—$A_1$, $A_2$,..., $A_n$, and to determine the time constants of restoration—$\tau_1$, $\tau_2$, ..., $\tau_n$. The plot of $1/\tau$ versus $A$ is *linear* as seen by reciprocating both sides of Equation (3.34):

$$1/\tau = k_1 A + k_2. \tag{3.36}$$

Thus, $k_1$ equals the slope and the $k_2$ equals the intercept.

Applications of the perturbation method to chemical equilibrium use two properties of equilibrium. First, equilibrium depends on external conditions such as temperature and pressure. For each temperature and pressure there is a particular set of forward and backward rate constants. Second, if an equilibrium is disturbed by changing the temperature or the pressure, the reaction cannot regain equilibrium infinitely fast. The restoration to equilibrium may, therefore, be monitored.

Tallarida and co-workers[40] in a theoretical paper considered the application of perturbation methods to pharmacological systems in equilibrium and later applied this method to the determination of $K$ for norepinephrine acting on isolated aortic strips of the rabbit.[41] The perturbing stimulus was ultraviolet light that was shown by Furchgott and co-workers to relax strips placed in a state of drug-induced contraction.[16] A basic assumption in this application is that ultraviolet upsets the equilibrium between drug and receptor. Although not directly proved, this assumption has support since the results of these experiments yielded a value of $K$ for norepinephrine that agrees with that determined by the method of partial irreversible blockage. Another line of supportive evidence is that the time constant for restoration is different in the presence of antagonists[23] in agreement with theoretical predictions.[39]

An excellent review of relaxation methods in chemistry is given by Larry Faller[12]; a more complete account is contained in the book by Czerlinski.[10]

*Example.* An isolated strip of rabbit aorta is contracted with a vasoconstricting drug in concentration $A_1 = 10^{-8}$ $M$. Upon reaching an equilibrium tension, ultraviolet photoflash is applied causing a brief loss of tension which recovers with time constant $\tau_1 = 35$ s. After recovery from the flash-induced relaxation, this same strip is given additional drug, bringing the total drug concentration to $A_2 = 10^{-6}$ $M$, and producing a new level of equilibrium tension. Ultraviolet flash is applied at this time causing less relaxation and a more rapid restoration given by the time constant $\tau_2 = 6$ s. From this experiment we can obtain the rate constants $k_1$ and $k_2$ for this drug by substituting in Equation (3.34): $35 = (k_1 10^{-8} + k_2)^{-1}$ and $6 = (k_1 10^{-6} + k_2)^{-1}$. Simultaneous solution yields $k_1 = 1.4 \times 10^5$ and $k_2 = 0.027$ from which $K = k_2/k_1 = 1.9 \times 10^{-7}$.*

## Allosteric Theory

It will be recalled that the fractional receptor binding $y$ of a drug is related to the drug concentration $A$ according to the relationship $y = A/(A + K)$, where $K$ is the dissociation constant. Also, a plot of $y$ versus $A$, using a linear scale of concentration, yields a hyperbolic curve. As this relation follows from the mass action law, it is no surprise that this kind of relation is seen in biological reactions other than those between a drug and a receptor. For example, oxygen binds to *myoglobin*, the oxygen-carrying protein of "red" muscle, according to such a relationship.

In contrast to myoglobin, the binding of oxygen to hemoglobin in blood results in a relation whose graph is sigmoidal or S-shaped when plotted with linear scales. In this situation the binding of $O_2$ to each of the four hemes is not independent of each other. The binding of one oxygen to heme is affected by the state of the other three hemes. The first oxygen binds relatively slowly, the second and third more rapidly, and the fourth binds very rapidly. This phenomenon is called *cooperativity* and has been shown to account for the S-shaped curve relating oxygen binding to hemoglobin. When applied to reactions between enzymes and substrates, cooperativity means that the combination of one substrate molecule to the enzyme enhances the affinity for the next substrate molecule. The enhancement may result from induced configurational changes in the enzyme, a so-called *allosteric* effect.[30,31]

The interest here in the allosteric theory results from the work of Changeux and co-workers[8] and of Karlin,[25] who extended allosteric theory to drug–receptor interactions. Working with agents that depolarize the electroplax cells of the eel, these investigators found a sigmoidal relation between the depolarization and the concentration. This relationship suggests cooperativity similar to that exhibited by the oxygen hemoglobin binding. (This is so if one assumes that depolarization is a satisfactory measure of drug effect.) Working with membrane conductance changes of the frog motor endplate induced by acetylcholine, Katz and Thesleff[26] and Jenkinson[24] found sigmoidal dose–response curves. These membrane effects of certain drugs have lent support for the allosteric theory in drug–receptor interactions.

In this theory it is postulated that the receptor exists in two conformational states which, in Karlin's terminology, are called R and T. The R form is the active

---

* Data from a *single* experiment for illustrative purposes only. See Jacob and Tallarida[23] and Tallarida et al.[41] for data obtained from a sample.

state and the T form is the inactive state. In the drug-free biological system these two forms are in equilibrium,

$$T \rightleftharpoons R$$

and the equilibrium ratio of the two forms is $L = T/R$. The constant $L$ is known as the allosteric constant. The basic mechanism is

$$A + R \underset{}{\overset{K_{AR}}{\rightleftharpoons}} AR$$
$$\Big\updownarrow$$
$$A + T \underset{K_{AT}}{\overset{}{\rightleftharpoons}} AT$$

Drugs act as agonists or antagonists according to their selective affinity for the R or T conformation, respectively.

This model of drug–receptor interaction is attractive because it provides a more detailed view of molecular events than does the occupation models of Clark, Ariëns, and Stephenson. It is reasonable to ask, however, how does the allosteric theory modify the values of the dissociation constants determined from the occupation theories?

It should be recalled that occupation theory provides methods for determining the dissociation constant $K$ for a strong agonist, a partial agonist, and a competitive antagonist. C. D. Thron[43] and D. Calquhoun,[7] acting independently, considered this question and arrived at essentially the same conclusion, viz., the allosteric model and the occupation model are experimentally indistinguishable in two cases: (1) the case of competitive antagonism and (2) the case in which a partial agonist is compared to a strong agonist. The drug–receptor dissociation constants determined by either method is that of the T form $K_{AT}$ or $K_{BT}$. Further, the efficacy, as defined by Stephenson,[36] depends, in allosteric theory, on the relative affinities of the drug for the R and T forms; i.e., the efficacy of an agonist is defined to be

$$\varepsilon_A = \frac{K_{AT}}{K_{AR}} - 1. \tag{3.37}$$

For an antagonist the efficacy is defined to be

$$\varepsilon_B = \frac{K_{BT}}{K_{BR}} - 1. \tag{3.38}$$

With this definition of efficacy both the allosteric model and the occupation model yield the same value for the dissociation constant of a partial agonist, as determined by the method of Equation (3.26), and for a competitive antagonist, as determined by the method of Equation (3.13). The $K$'s so determined are $K_{AT}$ and $K_{BT}$, respectively. It is only in the method of partial irreversible receptor inactivation that the two theories differ. In the occupation model this method leads to the relation given by Equation (3.24), with $K_A$ now taken to be $K_{AT}$:

$$\frac{1}{A} = \frac{1}{q} \cdot \frac{1}{A'} + \frac{1-q}{q} \cdot \frac{1}{K_{AT}}.$$

With the allosteric model the above no longer holds; instead we get

$$\frac{1}{A} = \frac{1}{q} \cdot \frac{1}{A'} + \frac{1-q}{q} \left( \frac{1}{K_{AT}} + \frac{1}{K_{AR}L} \right). \tag{3.39}$$

Thus, the allosteric model concludes that what is measured in the method of partial irreversible blockage is not $K_{AT}$, but $[K_{AT}^{-1} + (K_{AR}L)^{-1}]^{-1}$.

Apart from this difference, two other outcomes of allosteric theory are noteworthy. Both have to do with the definition of efficacy. First, the definition of efficacy allows for the possibility of negative efficacy. Second, this definition of efficacy allows for the possibility of nonparallel long-concentration response curves for competitive antagonism under certain conditions. The details of these arguments are not presented here; the reader is referred to the papers of Thron[43] and of Calquhoun.[7] As a summary statement we say only that the experimental evidence to date does not clearly favor one model over the other.

The validity of allosteric theory might be determined from a kind of experiment in which the $K$ of a weak agonist is determined in three ways.

Since the drug is a weak agonist it might be used as an *antagonist* to a full agonist which acts on the same receptor. The dissociation constant for the partial agonist can then be determined from the dose-ratio equation [Equation (3.13)]. Allosteric theory predicts that the $K$ so determined is that of the T form.

If this same drug is used as an *agonist*, and its agonistic action is compared to that of a full agonist acting on the same receptor, the method of Equation (3.26) may be used to determine its $K$. Again, allosteric theory predicts that the $K$ so determined is that of the T form.

When, however, the method of partial irreversible block is used (see p. 68), allosteric theory predicts that what is measured is not $K_{AT}$ but $(1/K_{AT} + 1/K_{AR}L)^{-1}$, a smaller quantity. Hence, of the three methods, allosteric theory says that the dissociation constant determined by partial irreversible blockade is smaller than that determined by the other two methods.

## Rate Theory

In contrast to the occupation theories that we have discussed, Professor W. D. M. Paton of Oxford has advanced a theory which assumes that the magnitude of a drug effect depends on the *rate of association* of drug and receptor.[33] The reaction

$$D + R \; \underset{k_2}{\overset{k_1}{\rightleftharpoons}} \; DR$$

is characterized by specific rate constants $k_1$ and $k_2$ for forward and reverse reactions. The properties of a drug thus depend on $k_1$, the association rate constant, and $k_2$ the dissociation rate constant. If $k_2$ is large, meaning that the drug readily leaves the receptor, then further association is possible. In this case the drug would be a strong agonist. A moderate value of $k_2$ means a partial agonist, and a low value of $k_2$ means that the drug is an antagonist. According to rate theory, therefore, an antagonist is a drug that leaves the receptor slowly. This theory also accounts for the persistence of effect of an antagonist on a tissue. Further, it accounts nicely for the phenomenon of "fade," i.e., the decline in the tissue response from its maximum, even though the drug concentration is not falling. Another feature of the rate theory is the possibility of determining the values of $k_1$ and $k_2$ for competitive antagonists from measurements of their rates of action. The rate of association for a drug in concentration $A$ is $k_1 A(r_t - x)$, where $x$ is the receptor occupancy. Since, at equilibrium, association rate, $k_1 A(r_t - x)$, equals dissociation rate, $k_2 X$, and since $x = r_t A/(A + k_2/k_1)$, the rate of association is

$$V_{\text{assoc}} = \frac{k_2 r_t A}{A + k_2/k_1}.$$

The response $E$ is taken to be directly proportional to association rate with proportionately constant $\phi$ (the same for all drugs). Thus, in rate theory, the equilibrium effect is

$$E = \frac{\phi k_2 r_t A}{A + k_2/k_1}. \tag{3.40}$$

Note the formal similarity between Equation (3.40) and Equation (3.7) of the classical occupation theory. In the latter, different drugs have different values of the constant $\alpha$. In Equation (3.40) different drugs have different values of the rate constant $k_2$, the value of $\phi$ being the same for all drugs acting on the receptor.

Equation (3.40) of rate theory demonstrates that the effect depends on $k_2$ as previously stated. It should be noted that $k_2/k_1$, the dissociation constant, is numerically equal to the $A_{50}$ concentration. This result is the same as that of the occupation model of classical theory (see p. 54).

An attractive feature of the rate theory is its simplicity. Efficacy differences of drugs are related to the differences in their values of $k_1$ and $k_2$; hence, there is no need for a third drug-dependent constant such as $\alpha$ in Equation (3.7). Also, rate theory provides a good explanation of the differences in rates of action between agonists and antagonists. This theory was tested by Paton on the guinea pig ileum using several different agonists and antagonists. The agreement was excellent. Yet in other systems there appears to be little support for the theory. Also several experimental results in the ileum, which are well explained by rate theory, can be equally well explained with other mechanisms. The details of the pros and cons of rate theory are nicely summarized in the review by Waud.[44]

For conditions short of equilibrium the rate of association is

$$V_{assoc} = \frac{Ar_t}{A + K} [k_2 + k_1 A \exp\{-(k_1 A + k_2)t\}].$$

The rate of association, therefore, is largest at $t = 0$ and decreases to its equilibrium value. This decline in $V_{assoc}$ accounts for the phenomenon of "fade" that was observed by Paton.

## References

1. Ariëns, E. J.: Arch. Int. Pharmacodynamie., 99:32, 1954.
2. Ariëns, E. J.: Molecular Pharmacology. New York, Academic Press, 1964.
3. Arunlakshana, O., and Schild, H. O.: Brit. J. Pharmacol., 14:48, 1959.
4. Barlow, R. B., Scott, N. C., and Stephenson, R. P.: Brit. J. Pharmacol. Chemother., 31:188, 1967.
5. Besse, J. C., and Furchgott, R. F.: J. Pharmacol. Exp. Ther., 197:66, 1976.
6. Broadley, K. J., and Nicholson, C. D.: Br. J. Pharmacol., 64:420P, 1978.
7. Calquhuon, D.: in Drug Receptors. (H. P. Rang, ed.) London, Macmillan, 1973, p. 149.
8. Changeux, J. P., Thiéry, J., Tung, Y., and Kittel, C.: Proc. U.S. Nat. Acad, Sci., 57:335, 1967.
9. Clark, A. J.: The Mode of Action of Drugs on Cells. Baltimore, Williams & Wilkins, 1933.
10. Czerlinski, G. H.: Chemical Relaxation. New York, Marcel Dekker, 1966.
11. Ehrlich, P.: in The collected papers of Paul Ehrlich. Vol. III: Chemotherapy. (F. Himmelweit, ed.), London, Pergamon Press, 1960.
12. Faller, L.: Sci. Am. May, 1969, p. 30.
13. Furchgott, R. F.: Ann. N.Y. Acad. Sci., 139:553, 1967.
14. Furchgott, R. F.: Fed. Proc., 37:115, 1978.
15. Furchgott, R. F., and Bursztyn, P.: Ann. N.Y. Acad. Sci., 144:882, 1967.
16. Furchgott, R. F., Ehrreich, S. J., and Greenblatt, E.: J. Gen. Physiol., 44:499, 1961.
17. Furchgott, R. F., Jurkiewicz, A., and Jurkiewicz, N. F.: in Frontiers of Catecholamine Research. (E. Usdin and S. Snyder, eds.) New York, Pergamon, 1973, p. 295.
18. Gaddum, J. H.: J. Physiol. (London), 89:7, 1937.
19. Gaddum, J. H.: Trans. Faraday Soc., 39:323, 1943.
20. Gero, A.: in Drill's Pharmacology in Medicine, 4th ed. (J. R. DiPalma, ed.) New York, McGraw-Hill, 1971, p. 71.
21. Gero, A.: J. Theor. Biol., 74:469, 1978.
22. Gero, A., and Tallarida, R. J.: J. Theor. Biol., 69:265, 1977.
23. Jacob, L. S., and Tallarida, R. J.: Arch. Int. Pharmacodynam., 225:166, 1977.
24. Jenkinson, D. H.: J. Physiol., 152:309, 1960.
25. Karlin, A. J.: Theoret. Biol., 16:306, 1967.
26. Katz, B., and Thesleff, S.: J. Physiol., 138:63, 1957.

27. Kenanin, T. P., and Black, J. W.: Mol. Pharmacol. *14*:607, 1978.
28. Langley, J. N.: J. Physiol. (London), *33*:374, 1905.
29. MacKay, D.: J. Pharm. Pharmacol., *30*:312, 1978.
30. Monod, J., Changeux, J. P., and Jacob, J.: J. Mol. Biol., *6*:306, 1963.
31. Monod, J., Wyman, J., and Changeux, J. P.: J. Mol. Biol., *12*:88, 1965.
32. Nickerson, M.: Nature, *178*:697, 1956.
33. Paton, W. D. M.: Proc. Roy. Soc. B., *154*:21, 1961.
34. Schild, H. O.: Brit. J. Pharmacol., *2*:189, 1947.
35. Sheys, E. M., and Green, R. D.: J. Pharmacol. Exp. Ther., *172*:320, 1970.
36. Stephenson, R. P.: Brit. J. Pharmacol., *11*:379, 1956.
37. Stone, M., and Angus, J. A.: J. Pharmacol. Exp. Ther., *207*:705, 1978.
38. Tallarida, R. J., Cowan, A., and Adler, M. W.: Life Sci., in press.
39. Tallarida, R. J., Laskin, O., and Jacob, L. S.: J. Theor. Biol., *61*:211, 1976.
40. Tallarida, R. J., Sevy, R. W., and Harakal, C.: Bull. Math. Biophysics., *32*:65, 1970.
41. Tallarida, R. J., Sevy, R. W., Harakal, C., and Loughnane, M.: IEEE Trans. Biomed. Engineering., *22*:493, 1975.
42. Tallarida, R. J., Sevy, R. W., Harakal, C., Bendrick, J., and Faust, R.: Arch. Int. Pharmacodynamie., *210*:67, 1974.
43. Thron, C. D.: Molec. Pharmacol., *9*:1, 1973.
44. Waud, D. R.: Pharm. Rev., *20*:49, 1968.
45. Waud, D. R.: J. Pharmacol. Exp. Ther., *170*:117, 1969.
46. Waud, D. R.: in *Methods in Pharmacology 3. Smooth Muscle.* (E. E. Daniel and D. M. Paton, eds.) New York, Plenum, 1975, chap. 27.

# Construction of Dose–Response Curves: Statistical Considerations

## Chapter 4

## Mean Dose and Mean Response

Biological systems demonstrate variability in their responses to drugs. Thus, the same muscle taken from two different animals (of the same species) and studied in vitro under controlled conditions will often give quantitatively different responses to identical doses of the same drug. Such variability is not unexpected since each muscle contains a large number of muscle fibers, and even the most careful surgical preparation of each is not likely to yield identical specimens. In addition to the variability in drug response that is due to slight differences in muscle composition or muscle orientation, there are other (unknown) factors that contribute to the variability. Indeed, there is generally even greater variability in drug responses in the whole animal, regardless of what response is measured. For these reasons we must use *mean* responses or average responses.

   The construction of dose–response curves, in particular the graded dose–response curve, is accomplished in two common statistical ways. In the first method, a fixed dose of drug is administered to the specimen and the given response is measured. Either the direct measure of the response can be used, or the response can be divided by the maximum response, yielding the relative response. If we multiply the relative response by 100, we get the percent response. Such a plot is shown in Figure 4.1. (This method of normalizing requires that the

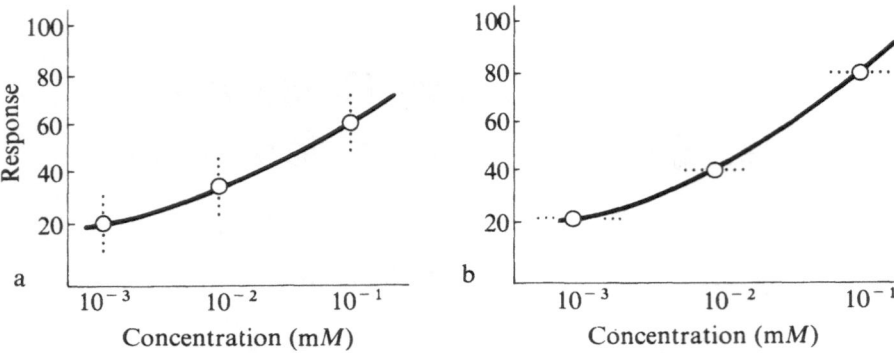

**Figure 4.1** Mean dose–response curves.

maximum response of the specimen be determined.) For example, Figure 4.1a illustrates the response in a set of specimens in each of which the maximum has been determined. It is seen that a dose of $10^{-3}$ mM gave responses ranging from 10% to 30% of the maximum, whereas $10^{-2}$ mM produced responses ranging from 20% to 50% of the maximum. For each dose the open circle is the mean response, expressed as a percent of the maximum. A smooth curve is drawn through the mean for each dose.

Another way of plotting is illustrated in Figure 4.1b. In this method, the range of concentrations necessary to produce a given response is plotted. The mean concentration for each effect is obtained and is indicated by the open circles. A smooth curve is drawn through these points. In general, the curves obtained from these two methods of plotting will be different. The linear portions of each will thus have different slopes. Ariëns et al.[1] point out that in many cases the slope of a curve obtained from the mean response to a given dose, of which Figure 4.1a is an example, is less than that obtained when mean concentration is used, as in Figure 4.1b. They further suggest that the second method (mean concentration) is the correct method. This suggestion is based on their observation that, of the two methods, the method of Figure 4.1b yields a slope which agrees more closely with theory. The theory that they use, however, assumes that the magnitude of the response is directly proportional to receptor occupancy, an assumption which is generally questionable (see p. 53). Hence, there is no convincing theoretical reason for preferring one method over the other. It might be pointed out, however, that the plot of Figure 4.1a, which uses mean response, is more easily attained experimentally.[2,4,6]

In each of the methods of plotting we have used the *mean* of a set of measured values. Other statistical concepts are important in the analysis of dose–response curves. We discuss these in the following sections. Although our immediate objective is the application of statistics to dose–response curves, the topics which follow represent a review of certain ideas in mathematical statistics that are applicable in general.

## Mean and Standard Deviation

A measurable characteristic, such as the tension in a muscle fiber, is called a *variable*. An individual measurement of a variable is called a *variate*. For the data of Figure 4.1, the variables are tension and dose, and the individual values of each are the variates. It is convenient to reduce a set of variates to a single measure which is descriptive of the set. Such a measure is the *arithmetic mean* (or, simply, *mean*) of a set of numbers $X_1, X_2, \ldots, X_N$. The mean, denoted by $\mu$, is defined as

$$\mu = \frac{X_1 + X_2 + \cdots + X_N}{N} = \frac{\sum_{i=1}^{N} X_i}{N}. \tag{4.1}$$

Of the $N$ variates $X_1, X_2, \ldots, X_N$, suppose some are equal so that there are only $L$ distinct numbers. Thus, we may have $X_1$ occur $f_1$ times, $X_2$ occur $f_2$ times, $\ldots$, $X_L$ occurs $f_L$ times. Then $f_1 + f_2 + \cdots + f_L = N$, and the mean becomes

$$\mu = \frac{X_1 f_1 + X_2 f_2 + \cdots + X_L f_L}{f_1 + f_2 + \cdots + f_2} = \frac{\sum_{i=1}^{N} X_i f_i}{N}. \tag{4.2}$$

The $\mu$ in Equation (4.2) is often called the *weighted mean* of the $L$ variates $X_1, X_2, \ldots, X_L$, since each of the variates is multiplied by its weight, or relative frequency, $f_i/N$.

The arithmetic mean is a useful measure of central tendency. It can sum up or describe a mass of data. Other measures of central tendency are also used. One such measure is the *median*. The median is the value of the middle item when an *odd* number of items are arranged in a nondecreasing sequence. For example, the set $\{4, 4, 5, 8, 12\}$ has a median of 5. When there is an even number of items in the (ordered) set, such as $\{5, 8, 12, 14, 15, 20\}$, the median is defined to be the arithmetic mean of the two central items. In the previous example, the median is 13, the mean of 12 and 14.

Other measures of central tendency are the *geometric mean*, the *harmonic mean*, and the *mode*. These are not very common in descriptions of dose-response relations and, therefore, will not be discussed here. The interested reader may find discussions of these in standard texts on statistics such as those mentioned in the references at the end of this chapter.

Although useful as measures of central tendency, the arithmetic mean and the median do not give information about the range of the variates or their dispersion. Thus, measures of the *deviations* of the set of variates about the mean are desirable. For example, the set $\{5, 6, 8, 10, 15, 16\}$ has a mean of 10, but so does the set $\{9, 10, 11\}$. Consider the first set. The difference between each variate and the mean, $X_i - \mu$, gives the set of deviations $\{-5, -4, -2, 0, 5, 6\}$. For the second set, the collection of deviations is $\{-1, 0, 1\}$. Note, in each case, the *sum of the deviations is zero*, a result which can easily be shown to apply always.

Hence, the sum of deviations from the mean is not a useful indication of the degree of dispersion. If the *magnitudes* of the deviations are added, however, we do get a useful measure of dispersion. Division of this sum by the number of variates $N$ gives the *mean deviation*, denoted by M.D.:

$$\text{M.D.} = \frac{\sum_{i=1}^{N} |X_i - \mu|}{N}. \tag{4.2'}$$

For the two sets above the mean deviations are 22/6 and 2/3. We see, therefore, that the mean deviation discriminates adequately between these two sets that have the same mean.

Since the square of any real number is nonnegative, the sum of the squared deviations from the mean can also serve as a measure of dispersion. If this sum is divided by the number of items in the set, we obtain a quantity called the *variance* which we shall denote by the symbol $\sigma^2$. Thus,

$$\sigma^2 = \frac{\sum_{i=1}^{N} (X_i - \mu)^2}{N}. \tag{4.3}$$

The square root of the variance is the *standard deviation* $\sigma$, a widely used measure of dispersion. Thus,

$$\sigma = \sqrt{\frac{\sum_{i=1}^{N} (X_i - \mu)^2}{N}}. \tag{4.4}$$

*Example.* Given the set $\{4.5, 4.0, 5.0, 4.2, 4.7, 5.5, 5.2\}$ find the standard deviation. The mean is 4.7. Thus

$$\sigma = \sqrt{\frac{(4.5 - 4.7)^2 + (4.0 - 4.7)^2 + \cdots + (5.2 - 4.7)^2}{7}}$$

$$= 0.50.$$

## Samples and Populations

In collecting dose–response data and, indeed, in most research work, we are interested in the data because they may represent some other, larger set of data. For example, when we determine the response developed in a set of 10 mice in response to a particular dose of some stimulating drug, we are determining a measure in a *sample* in order to learn about this same response in a *population*. The totality of the measurements obtained from *all* mice of the same strain, age, and weight constitutes the population. The mean and standard deviation discussed previously are *population parameters*. In the previous example the set of measurements constituted the whole population. In most instances, however, we can only work with a sample from the population. Quantities calculated from a sample, such as the mean and the standard deviation, are called *statistics*.

In order to distinguish the population parameters, mean ($\mu$) and standard deviation ($\sigma$), from the corresponding *sample mean* and *standard deviation*, we shall use the notation $\bar{x}$ for the sample mean and $s$ for the sample standard deviation. The *sample mean* of a set of variates $X_1, X_2, \ldots, X_N$ is given by a formula identical to that of Equation (4.1):

$$\bar{X} = (\textstyle\sum^N X_i)/N.$$

However, the *standard deviation of a sample* is defined as

$$s = \sqrt{\frac{\sum^N (X_i - \bar{X})^2}{N - 1}}. \tag{4.5}$$

The *sample variance* is then denoted by $s^2$, and is given by

$$s^2 = \frac{\sum_{i=1} (X_i - \bar{X})^2}{N - 1}. \tag{4.6}$$

The reason for division by $N - 1$ for a sample and $N$ for a population will not be discussed here. We should note, however, that, for sufficiently large values of $N$, the difference is not important.

## Distributions

When discussing the mean of a set of $N$ variates, we considered the case in which the variate $x_1$ occurred $f_1$ times, $x_2$ occurred $f_2$ times, $\ldots$, $x_L$ occurred $f_L$ times. In this situation the numbers $x_i$ are variates of a *discrete* random variable. Examples of discrete variables are the number of cases of measles among a population of school children, or the number of individuals who receive polio vaccinations in a given year. If a variable can assume *any* value between certain limits, it is called a *continuous* variable. Examples of continuous variables are those representing weight, height, and blood pressure. For a discrete variable we take the number or frequency of occurrence for each value of the variable, thus producing a *frequency distribution*. For a continuous variable we must dissect the range of the variable into intervals or *class boundaries*. The frequency distribution in this case gives the number of times the variable is contained within the class boundary. *Relative frequency*, i.e., the number divided by the total number, may be used instead of frequency for either the discrete or the continuous variable.

It is convenient to display frequency distributions. Usually the variable is shown on the abscissa and the frequency on the ordinate. For displaying

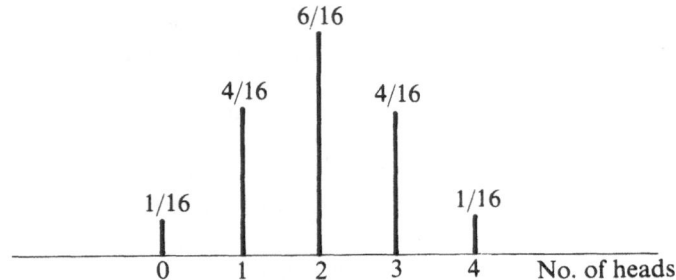

**Figure 4.2** Four coins are tossed simultaneously. The height of the vertical line is the theoretical relative frequency of occurrence of the number of heads shown on the abscissa.

a discrete variable such as the outcome of a coin toss a simple diagram consisting of vertical lines might be used, as in Figure 4.2. For continuous variables such as the weights of a population of laboratory animals, the variates are grouped within defined class boundaries, and a vertical bar chart or *histogram* is constructed, as in Figure 4.3. In this example, the class interval 49–54 includes all variates that are between 48.5 and 54.5. The midpoint is 51.5. The next class interval, 55–60, includes all that are between 54.5 and 60.5. In this case the midpoint is 57.5. The midpoints are used in the calculation of the arithmetic mean. Thus,

$$\mu = \frac{(5)(51.5) + (15)(57.5) + (23)(63.5) + (35)(69.5) + (22)(75.5)}{5 + 15 + 23 + 35 + 22} = 66.7.$$

The variance is computed using the midpoint $x_i$ of the $i$th interval:

$$\sigma^2 = \frac{\sum f_i(x_i - \mu)^2}{\sum f_i}. \tag{4.7}$$

If the amount of data were very large, and if we chose very small class intervals, the resulting histogram would take on the appearance of a region whose upper boundary would look like a smooth curve called a distribution. Examples of distribution curves are shown in Figure 4.4.

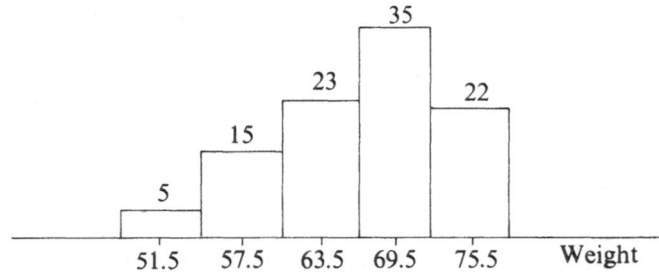

**Figure 4.3** Histogram for the weights of 100 laboratory animals. The mean is 66.7. The variance $\sigma^2$, computed from Equation (4.7), is 46.4, yielding $\sigma = 6.81$.

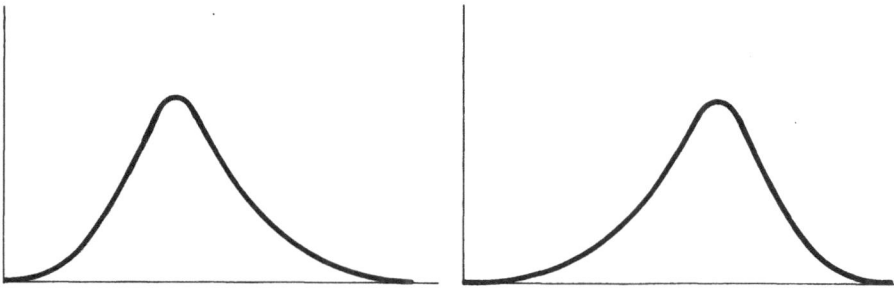

**Figure 4.4** Distribution curves.

## Normal Distribution

A distribution curve of great importance in statistics is shown in Figure 4.5. If we take a *large* sample of some variable such as the systolic blood pressures of American men, and draw a histogram with small class intervals, the shape will be very much like the curve of Figure 4.5. This symmetric, bell-shaped curve represents a *normal* distribution. The axis of symmetry of the curve is at the mean of the sample. The normal curve will be different for samples drawn from different populations; for example, men's weights will give a different curve than that for their blood pressures. Also, men's weights will give a different curve than women's weights. These normal curves will have different heights, different means, and different widths, yet a symmetrical bell-shaped distribution curve

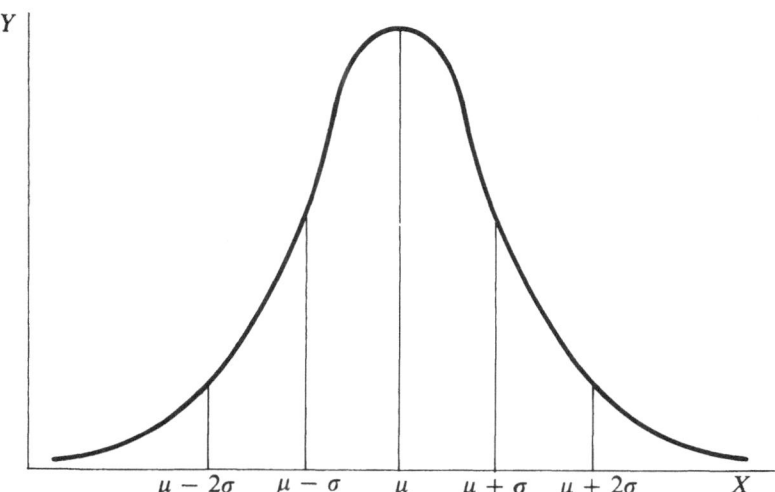

**Figure 4.5** The normal curve.

will describe the distribution of each of these variables. One usually constructs the histogram by plotting the *relative frequency* rather than the frequency on the ordinate. The relative frequency is merely the ratio of the number of variates having a particular value to the total number. The term "probability" is used for the theoretical relative frequency, the latter being the limit as the size of the sample increases without bound. When the relative frequency is plotted in a histogram for a large amount of data using very small class intervals, the smooth distribution curve is called the *normal frequency curve*, or *normal curve*. The equation of the normal curve is

$$Y = \frac{1}{\sigma\sqrt{2\pi}} \exp\left[-\frac{(x - \mu)^2}{2\sigma^2}\right]. \tag{4.7'}$$

The total area between the normal curve and the $x$ axis is 1 square unit, regardless of the values of $\mu$ and $\sigma$. Thus, *the area under the curve between points $x_1$ and $x_2$ is equal to the expected proportion of cases that fall between these points.* Put another way, the area between $x_1$ and $x_2$ is the probability that $x$ is between $x_1$ and $x_2$. It is therefore important to be able to measure these areas. There are, however, an infinite number of normal curves, one for each pair $(\mu, \sigma)$. In order to tabulate areas for any particular normal curve, we use the *standard normal curve* obtained from the transformation

$$Z = \frac{x - \mu}{\sigma}. \tag{4.8}$$

This transformation results in a recalibration of the abscissa in terms of $Z$, as shown in Figure 4.6. Note that $x = \mu$ corresponds to $Z = 0$; $x = \mu + \sigma$ corresponds to $Z = 1$, and $x = \mu - \sigma$ corresponds to $Z = -1$, etc. The unit along the $Z$-axis is $\sigma$, the standard deviation of the variable $x$.

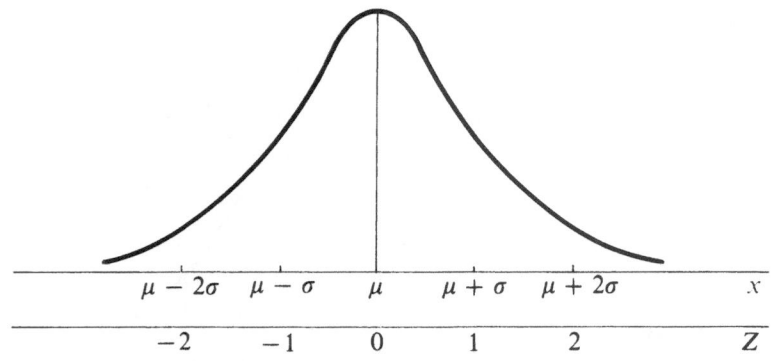

**Figure 4.6** Conversion to standard units $Z$.

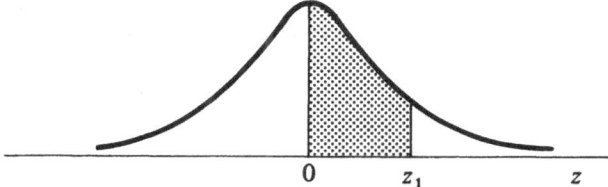

**Figure 4.7** Area under the standard normal curve.

The area under the standard normal curve is obtained from a table. Because the curve is symmetric, it is only necessary to tabulate the area for positive values of $Z$. The entry corresponding to a given value of $Z$, say $Z_1$, is the area between $Z = 0$ and $Z = Z_1$, shown shaded in Figure 4.7.

If, for example, it is desired to determine the area between $Z = -2$ and $Z = -1$, we find the area between $Z = +1$ and $Z = +2$. This area is determined as the difference of the areas, Area($Z = 2$) $-$ Area($Z = 1$), as shown in Figure 4.8. Note

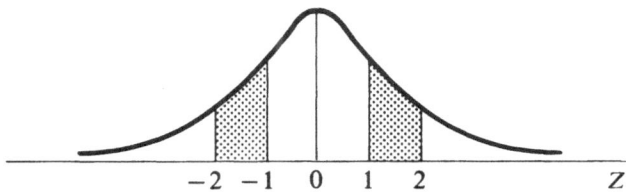

**Figure 4.8** Determination of area between $Z = -2$ and $Z = -1$.

that the tabular entry for $Z = 1$ is, from Table A.1, 0.3413. Since $Z = 1$ corresponds to $x = \mu + \sigma$, we see that the area contained within one standard deviation on either side of the mean is $2 \times 0.3413 = 0.6826$. Hence, about 68 % of the area is contained within $\mu \pm \sigma$. From the entry for $Z = 2$ we see that about 95 % of the area is contained within $\mu + 2\sigma$ (Fig. 4.9).

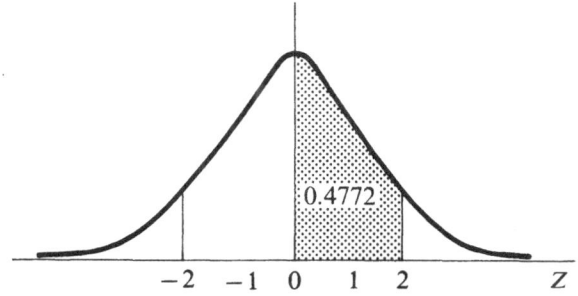

**Figure 4.9** Area contained within $\mu \pm 2\sigma \approx 95 \%$ of the area.

*Example.* The weights of a certain strain of adult male rabbits are approximately normally distributed; further, the mean weight is 2.6 kg and the standard deviation of the weights is 0.3 kg. What proportion of these animals have weights greater than 3 kg?

Changing scales, we have $Z = (x - 2.6)/(0.3)$. For $x = 3.0$ kg, $Z = (3.0 - 2.6)/(0.3) = 1.3$. From Table A.1, the area between $Z = 0$ and $Z = 1.3$ is 0.403. The total area to the left of $Z = 0$ is 0.500. Hence, $0.500 + 0.403 = 0.903$ gives the proportion of weights that are less than or equal to 3 kg. The difference, $1 - 0.903 = 0.097$, is the proportion greater than 3 kg.

This example demonstrates the convenience of the standard normal distribution. We did not need detailed information about the shape of the distribution for the population of rabbit weights. Having the values of $\mu$ and $\sigma$ was sufficient. In many cases, however, we do not know $\mu$ and $\sigma$. In such cases, we take a sample of size $n$ and determine the sample mean $\bar{X}$ and the sample standard deviation $s$. If we take repeated samples of size $n$ from a normally distributed population we get a set of sample means: $\bar{x}_1, \bar{x}_2, \ldots$ . *The set of means are normally distributed.* This set gives the *distribution of sample means*, and the *mean of the population of sample means is the same as the mean of the original population.* The mean of the samples will be denoted by $\mu_{\bar{x}}$. Hence,

$$\mu_{\bar{x}} = \mu. \tag{4.9}$$

The standard deviation of the distribution of samples, denoted by $\sigma_{\bar{x}}$, is *not* the same as $\sigma$. It can be shown that these are related as

$$\sigma_{\bar{x}} = \frac{\sigma}{\sqrt{n}}. \tag{4.10}$$

In other words, $\sigma_{\bar{x}}$ is smaller than $\sigma$, a fact which is reasonable since the set of sample means has less dispersion than the set of variates of the population.

Even if the *parent population is not normally distributed,* the set of sample means will approach a normal distribution as *n gets large.* Equations (4.9) and (4.10) are still applicable in this case. The standard deviation of the set of sample means, denoted previously by $\sigma_{\bar{x}}$, is often called the *standard error of the mean* (abbreviated S.E.M.).

## Estimation

*Estimation* is a process whereby we infer some unknown attribute of a population, such as its mean, by determining the corresponding attribute from a random sample drawn from that population. Thus, whenever we determine the mean response to a specific dose of a drug in some species we are working with a sample. The mean so determined is an estimate of the population mean. It is intuitively clear that the size of the sample should be sufficiently large if we are to have reasonable confidence in the estimate.

In the previous section, we saw that for a sufficiently large sample the sampling distribution of the mean is approximately normal, with standard deviation $= \sigma/\sqrt{n}$ and mean $= \mu$. Often we do not know $\sigma$, but if $n \geq 30$, we can use $s$, the sample standard deviation. In this case $\sigma_{\bar{x}}$ becomes $s/\sqrt{n}$. The standard variate in this case is

$$Z = \frac{\bar{x} - \mu}{\sigma_{\bar{x}}} = \frac{\bar{x} - \mu}{s/\sqrt{n}}.$$

From Table A.1 we see that 95 % of the area under the normal curve lies between the interval $|Z| < 1.96$. Hence

$$\left| \frac{\bar{x} - \mu}{s/\sqrt{n}} \right| < 1.96$$

gives the 95 % *confidence interval for the mean*. Rewriting the inequality without the absolute values gives

$$\bar{x} - 1.96 \frac{s}{\sqrt{n}} < \mu < \bar{x} + 1.96 \frac{s}{\sqrt{n}}. \tag{4.11}$$

*Example.* A sample of 40 aortic strips stimulated with $10^{-7} M$ phenylephrine produced a mean tension of 4.5 g with standard deviation 0.3 g. The 95 % confidence interval is $4.5 \pm (1.96)(0.3)/\sqrt{40} = 4.5 \pm 0.093$ g. The 99 % *confidence interval may be determined* from the values of $Z$ between which 99 % of the area lies. From Table A.1 we see that this value is $Z = 2.58$. Hence, the 99 % confidence interval is $4.5 \pm (2.58)(0.3)/\sqrt{40} = 4.5 \pm 0.122$ g.

A common practice when plotting dose–response curves or tabulating dose–response data is to indicate the mean response $\bar{x} \pm$ the standard error of the mean $(s/\sqrt{n})$ for each dose. Multiplication of the standard error by the appropriate value of $Z$ (1.96 for 95 % or 2.58 for 99 %) gives the confidence interval.

When the parent population is believed to be normally distributed and the sample size $n \geq 30$, one can use the normal distribution in order to get confidence limits for the population mean $\mu$ from the statistics $\bar{x}$ and $s$ as previously shown [Equation (4.11)]. When, however, the sample size is *small* it is necessary to use the "$t$" distribution. This distribution, like the normal distribution, is symmetric, although its dispersion is somewhat greater. As $n$ increases the $t$ distribution approaches in shape the normal distribution. Values of $t$ correspond to areas under this symmetric curve, just as values of $Z$ give areas under the standard normal curve. Unlike the standard normal curve which is unique, the

$t$ distribution is not unique. Its use, as seen from Table A.2 requires the use of "degrees of freedom," denoted here by the symbol "$v$," and the prior specification of the area under the curve (probability). In the $t$ table the probabilities are usually listed across the top. In Table A.2 three probabilities are used: 90%, 95%, and 99%. The degrees of freedom $v$ are listed down the first column. For example, corresponding to $p = 95\%$ and $v = 10$, we see that $t = 2.228$. The value of $v$, as we shall see, is related to the sample size $n$, and the number of parameters being estimated. In the estimation problem under consideration, we are interested in the estimate of the mean $\mu$. In this case, $v = n - 1$.

The formula for $t$ resembles that for $Z$:

$$t = \frac{\bar{x} - \mu}{s/\sqrt{n}}. \tag{4.12}$$

From Equation (4.12), it follows that a confidence interval for $\mu$ is determined from

$$\bar{x} \pm (t)(s/\sqrt{n}) \tag{4.13}$$

where $t$ is determined with $n - 1$ degrees of freedom and the desired degree of confidence. Thus, if a 95% confidence interval is desired and the sample size $n = 10$, we find from the table that $t = 2.262$ corresponding to 9 degrees of freedom. From Equation (4.13) the 95% confidence interval is $\bar{x} \pm 2.262\, s/\sqrt{10}$.

The $t$ distribution is widely used in estimating mean responses to drugs since in many laboratory situations the sample size is small. Commonly we get the mean response to a particular dose by administering this dose to, say, 10 specimens, followed by a different (higher dose) to another 10 specimens, etc. For each dose the mean response and its standard error $s/\sqrt{10}$ is found. Multiplying the standard error by the appropriate $t$ value, as in Equation (4.13), yields the confidence interval of response for each dose.

*Example.* Two doses, 2 and 8 mg/kg of morphine sulfate, are administered s.c. to two different groups of 15 rats. The mean responses, analgesia (as a percent of maximum), 39 min after administration are given below along with the standard error of the mean. From Table A.2, $t_{95} = 2.145$.

| Dose | Mean response (S.E.M.) |
|------|------------------------|
| 2    | 32 (5)                 |
| 8    | 81 (4)                 |

The half-widths of the 95% confidence intervals are $(2.145)(5)/\sqrt{15} = 2.77$, for the 2 mg/kg dose, and $(2.145)(4)/\sqrt{15} = 2.21$ for the 8 mg/kg dose. The confidence intervals may be written $32 \pm 2.8$ and $81 \pm 2.2$ when rounded to two significant figures.

## Tests of Significance

If a drug is administered to one group of subjects while another group receives an inert substance (placebo), we can apply statistical methods in order to determine whether the responses in each group *differ significantly*. Put another way, if we compare the mean responses of the groups, what is the probability that the difference in means is due to chance? The investigator must specify, therefore, the probability that he is willing to accept in answering this question. If the probability ($P$) selected is, say, 0.05, we say that the difference in the means is significant "at the level 0.05." If we desire greater significance then we must specify a lower probability such as 0.01 or 0.001.

Our interest, of course, is in determining whether the means of the two populations ($\mu_1$ and $\mu_2$) differ, one population being the drug group and the other the placebo group. As usual, we take samples, yielding means $\bar{X}_1$ and $\bar{X}_2$ and standard deviations $s_1$ and $s_2$. The hypothesis being tested is that $\mu_1 - \mu_2 = 0$, a *null* hypothesis. Now the sampling distribution of the statistic $\bar{X}_1 - \bar{X}_2$ has the mean $\mu_1 - \mu_2$ and the standard deviation

$$\sigma_{\bar{X}_1 - \bar{X}_2} = \sqrt{\frac{\sigma_1^2}{n_1} + \frac{\sigma_2^2}{n_2}} \tag{4.14}$$

where $n_1$ and $n_2$ are the respective sample sizes. For sufficiently large samples (e.g., $n_1 \geq 30$ and $n_2 \geq 30$) the distribution $\bar{X}_1 - \bar{X}_2$ is approximately normal and the sample standard deviations $s_1$ and $s_2$ can be taken for $\sigma_1$ and $\sigma_2$. Thus, we form the statistic

$$Z = \frac{\bar{X}_1 - \bar{X}_2}{\sqrt{(s_1^2/n_1) + (s_2^2/n_2)}} \tag{4.15}$$

which has approximately the standard normal distribution. Having specified the probability $P$ that the null hypothesis is true (i.e., that $\mu_1 = \mu_2$), we now compare the $Z$ value computed from Equation (4.15) with the $Z$ obtained from our specified probability. For example, if we specify $P = 0.01$, the $Z$ from Table A.1 is 2.58. Hence, if the value calculated from Equation (4.15) is *equal to or greater than* 2.58, *we reject the null hypothesis* and conclude that the *means are significantly different* with $P \leq 0.01$.

When the *sample sizes are small* (i.e., either $n_1$ or $n_2$ less than 30), we apply the above reasoning with the employment of the $t$ distribution discussed previously, provided that the parent *populations are approximately normal* with equal standard deviation $\sigma_1$ and $\sigma_2$. In terms of the small sample sizes $n_1$ and $n_2$ and the sample statistics $\bar{X}_1, \bar{X}_2, s_1$ and $s_2$, we compute $t$ for degrees of freedom $v = n_1 + n_2 - 2$ from the formula

$$t = (\bar{X}_1 - \bar{X}_2) \Big/ \left( \sqrt{\frac{(n_1 - 1)s_1^2 + (n_2 - 1)s_2^2}{n_1 + n_2 - 2}} \sqrt{\frac{1}{n_1} + \frac{1}{n_2}} \right) \tag{4.16}$$

As in the large-sample test, the value of $t$ must equal or exceed the tabular value for the specified criteria in terms of $P$ if the difference is to be significant. In pharmacological testing we ordinarily take $P = 0.05$ or $P = 0.01$.

> *Example.* The observation was made that a new drug being tested increased the heart rate in dogs. It was decided to determine whether this action was dose related. To this end, six dogs were injected with 10 mg/kg of the drug and experienced an average increase in heart rate of 20 beats/min, with a standard deviation of 2.8 beats/min. Eight dogs who received the larger dose, 50 mg/kg, experienced an average increase in rate of 27 beats/min, with a standard deviation of 3.5 beats/min.
>
> In order to determine whether these mean responses differ significantly, we employ the $t$ test from Equation (4.16) because the sample sizes are small. Using $\bar{X}_1 = 20$, $\bar{X}_2 = 27$, $s_1 = 2.8$, $s_2 = 3.5$, $n_1 = 6$, and $n_2 = 8$, we get
>
> $$t = (20 - 27)\Bigg/ \sqrt{\frac{5(2.8)^2 + 7(3.5)^2}{12}}\ \sqrt{\frac{1}{6} + \frac{1}{8}}$$
>
> $$= -4.02.$$

Since this value of $t$ exceeds in magnitude the tabular entry 2.179 for 95% ($P = 0.05$) and 12 degrees of freedom, the difference in the means is significant. In fact, the tabular value for 99% is 3.055. Hence, this difference is significant with $P < 0.01$.

## Linear Regression

There are many situations in which theory predicts that a linear relation should exist between two variables, $x$ and $y$; yet, when the actual data are plotted, the points are not colinear. Also, we meet situations in which no a priori assumption of linearity exists but, when the pairs $(x_i, y_i)$ are plotted, there is a basic linear trend. In either case we have a set of plotted points as in Figure 4.10 to which we wish to fit a line. This process of fitting a line is called *linear regression*.

One might attempt to draw "by eye" a straight line that represents the trend. It is likely, however, that no two individuals would draw exactly the same line. Thus, we need an *objective* method for fitting the line to the observed $n$ variates $(x_i, y_i)$. Such an objective method is that known as *least squares*. In the method of least squares we apply the criterion that the line of best fit is that which minimizes the sum of the squares of the vertical distances from the points to the line. Figure 4.10 shows these vertical distances or deviations. If we denote by $\hat{y}_i$ the ordinate on the line, and by $y_i$ the observed value of $y$, then the deviation is $d_i = \hat{y}_i - y_i$, and the squared deviation is $(\hat{y}_i - y_i)^2$. The least squares criterion requires that the sum, $\sum_{i=1}^{n} (\hat{y}_i - y_i)^2$, should be as small as possible. We now discuss the method for finding the equation of this line. Since the slope-intercept equation of the line is $y = mx + b$, the objective of the method is to determine

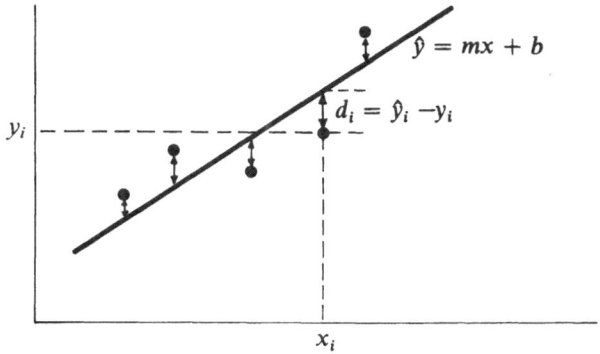

**Figure 4.10** Vertical deviation from the point $(x_i, y_i)$ to the line.

$m$ and $b$ for the best fitting line. It should be noted that the line that we obtain may *not contain* any of the plotted points. The line will, however, contain the point $(\bar{x}, \bar{y})$, where $\bar{x}$ and $\bar{y}$ are the respective arithmetic means of the sets $\{x_i\}$ and $\{y_i\}$. Hence, an alternate way of expressing the least squares line is the *point-slope form* (see p. 25):

$$\hat{y} - \bar{y} = m(x - \bar{x}). \tag{4.17}$$

It can be shown (using the techniques of calculus) that the slope $m$ is given by

$$m = \frac{\sum y_i(x_i - \bar{x})}{\sum (x_i - \bar{x})^2}. \tag{4.18}$$

The $y$-intercept $b$ is given by

$$b = \bar{y} - m\bar{x}. \tag{4.19}$$

The numbers $m$ and $b$ are called *regression coefficients* in the statistical literature. Since $m$ and $b$ are statistics, it is desirable to determine the standard error (and *confidence interval*) of each. Details of such an analysis are not presented here. We give only the formulas and refer the interested reader to the several references listed at the end of this chapter.

The standard errors (S.E.) of slope $(m)$, $y$-intercept $(b)$, and $x$-intercept $(x^*)$ are given by

$$\text{S.E.}(m) = s_e \left[ \frac{1}{\sum (x_i - \bar{x})^2} \right]^{1/2} \tag{4.20}$$

$$\text{S.E.}(b) = s_e \left[ \frac{1}{n} + \frac{(\bar{x})^2}{\sum (x_i - \bar{x})^2} \right]^{1/2} \tag{4.21}$$

and

$$\text{S.E.}(x^*) = \left| \frac{s_e}{m} \right| \cdot \left[ \frac{1}{n} + \frac{(\bar{y}/b)^2}{\sum (x_i - \bar{x})^2} \right]. \tag{4.22}$$

In each of these equations $n$ is the number of points and $s_e$, called the *standard error of estimate*, is obtained from

$$s_e^2 = \frac{\sum (\hat{y}_i - y_i)^2}{n - 2}. \tag{4.23}$$

Confidence intervals for the parameters are obtained by multiplying the standard error by either $Z$ (large sample) or $t$ (small sample) for the appropriate degree of confidence (usually 95% or 99%). In most pharmacological experiments, we are dealing with a small sample ($n < 30$); hence, we most often use the $t$ distribution with ($n - 2$) *degrees of freedom*.

*Example.* In a study of the vasoconstrictor action of phenylephrine on isolated rabbit aorta, the concentration–response data in columns 1 and 2 were obtained.[19] Find the regression line and the 95% confidence interval of the slope.

| Log (molar conc.) = $x$ | Response (% of max) = $y$ | $\hat{y}$ (from regression line) |
|---|---|---|
| −7.5 | 18 | 18.5 |
| −7.4 | 28 | 27.2 |
| −7.2 | 43 | 44.5 |
| −7.1 | 55 | 53.2 |
| −6.9 | 70 | 70.6 |

For these data: $\bar{x} = -7.22$, $\bar{y} = 42.8$. The equation of the regression line is $\hat{y} = 86.8x + 669$, as shown below. From Equation (4.18), the slope is

$$m = \frac{(18)(-7.5 + 7.22) + \cdots + (70)(-6.9 + 7.22)}{(-7.5 + 7.22)^2 + \cdots + (-6.9 + 7.22)^2}$$

$$= 86.8.$$

From Equation (4.19), the intercept is

$$b = 42.8 - 86.8(-7.22)$$
$$= 669.$$

Hence, the equation of the regression line is

$$\hat{y} = 86.8x + 669. \tag{4.24}$$

From the regression equation we can calculate the ordinate on the line, $\hat{y}$, corresponding to each $x$ by substitution of the $x_i$ into Equation (4.24). The results are tabulated in column 3. The quantity $s_e^2$ is computed from Equation (4.23):

$$s_e^2 = \frac{(18.5 - 18)^2 + (27.2 - 28)^2 + (44.5 - 43)^2 + (53.2 - 55)^2 + (70.6 - 70)^2}{5 - 2}$$

$$= 2.25.$$

Thus $s_e = 1.50$. The reader may verify that substitution into Equation (4.20) yields S.E.$(m) = 3.15$. The 95% confidence interval is obtained by multiplying 3.15 by the $t$ value for 3 degrees of freedom. From the $t$ table, this value is 3.182. Hence, the 95% confidence interval of the slope is $86.8 \pm (3.15)(3.182) = 86.8 \pm 10.0$. The graph is shown in Figure 4.11.

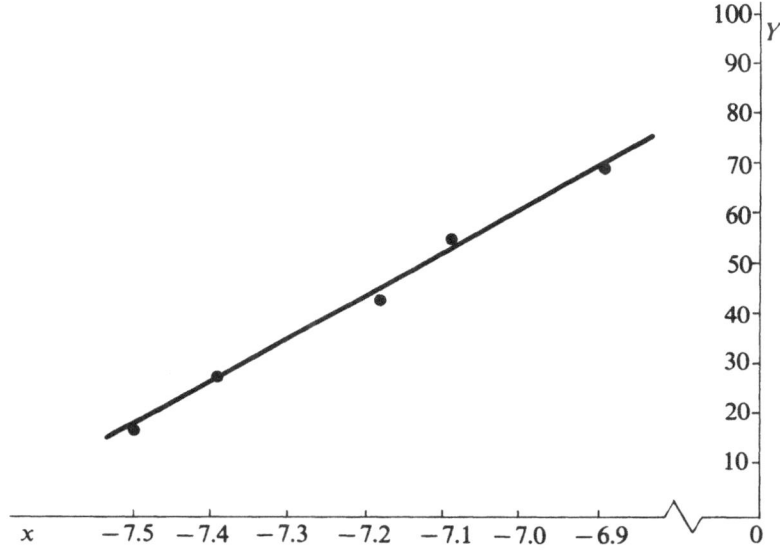

**Figure 4.11** Regression line.

*Example.* In order to determine the $pA_2$ of an antagonist drug a Schild plot was made as in Figure 4.12 (see p. 64). We wish to determine the $x$-intercept and its 95% confidence interval. In a Schild plot, the dose-ratio $(dr)$ of agonist is determined in the presence of a fixed concentration $(B)$ of antagonist. The ordinate $y = \log(dr - 1)$; the abscissa $x = -\log B$. In the graph of Figure 4.12 the units

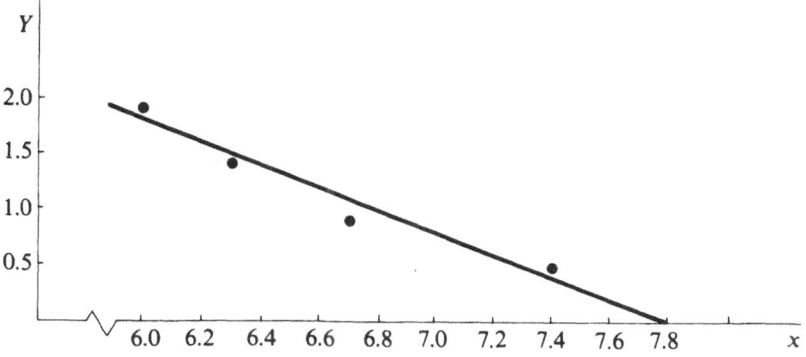

**Figure 4.12** The Schild plot.

of $B$ are molar. Hence, the $pA_2$ is obtained directly from the $x$-intercept. The points $(x, y)$ are $(6, 1.9)$, $(6.3, 1.4)$, $(6.7, 0.9)$, and $(7.4, 0.5)$. The regression equation for this line is $\hat{y} = -0.97x + 7.6$. The $pA_2 = 7.8$. Application of Equation (4.22) to these data gave S.E.$(x) = 0.098$. Multiplying 0.098 by the value of $t$ for 2 degrees of freedom ($t = 4.30$ from Table A.2) yields 0.42. Hence, the 95% interval for the $pA_2$ is $7.8 \pm 0.42$.

For theoretical reasons we sometimes want the regression line to have *unit slope*. In this case we are fitting the points, not to the best straight line, but to the best straight line of slope 1. The equation of the regression line is, therefore, $\hat{y} = x + b$. There is just one constant to determine, namely, $b$, the $y$-intercept. It can be shown that $b$ is given by

$$b = \frac{\sum (y_i - x_i)}{n} \tag{4.25}$$

for the $n$ data points $(x_i, y_i)$. For a line of *slope* $-1$, the equation for the intercept is

$$b = \frac{\sum (y_i + x_i)}{n}. \tag{4.26}$$

This type of *constrained* plot is a theoretical requirement of the Schild plot (see the previous example and p. 64). For the data of the previous example, application of Equation (4.26) gives

$$b = \frac{(6 + 1.9) + (6.3 + 1.4) + (6.7 + 0.9) + (7.4 + 0.5)}{4} = 7.775,$$

or, by rounding, 7.8. This value agrees well with the value 7.8 previously determined. Of course, in cases in which the slope of the regression line is very different from unity, the intercepts determined by each method will be correspondingly different.

The *goodness of fit* of the regression line to the $n$ points $(x_i, y_i)$ is measured by the *correlation coefficient $r$*, given by the formula

$$r = \frac{\sum (y_i - \bar{y})(x_i - \bar{x})}{[\sum (y_i - \bar{y})^2 \sum (x_i - \bar{x})^2]^{1/2}} \tag{4.27}$$

or the more convenient computational formula

$$r = \frac{\sum x_i y_i - n\bar{x}\bar{y}}{[(\sum x_i^2 - n\bar{x}^2)(\sum y_i^2 - n\bar{y}^2)]^{1/2}}. \tag{4.28}$$

The correlation coefficient is always a number in the interval $-1 \leq r \leq 1$. If $r = +1$ or $r = -1$, *then all points lie on the line*. If $r$ is "close to" $+1$ or $-1$, a good linear relationship exists. If $r = 0$, no linear relation exists between $x$

and $y$. The sign of $r$ is the same as that of the slope of the line. The reader can verify that the correlation coefficient in the first example (p. 100) is 0.998, indicative of a strong linear relationship between $x$ (log dose) and $y$ (response). For the Schild plot in the second example, $r = -0.97$.

## Parallel Lines—Assays and Antagonism

The potency of an agonist is frequently determined by comparison with the potency of some standard agonist having similar action. For example, in Figure 4.13 the responses $E$ to agonist 1 (the standard) and agonist 2 (the unknown) are plotted as functions of log dose. Although the dose–response plots are not linear over the entire ranges of doses, we frequently find a region of linearity. In order to compare potency we may require that the curves be parallel. Parallel log dose–response curves are also a theoretical requirement when a fixed dose of a competitive antagonist is administered along with the agonist.

If the departure from parallelism is not too great, we take the common slope $m$ to be the *weighted* mean of the slopes. Thus, if $m_1$ is the slope of line 1 and $m_2$ is the slope of line 2 (each determined by least squares), we have

$$m = \frac{w_1 m_1 + w_2 m_2}{w_1 + w_2} \tag{4.29}$$

where the weight $w_i$ of each is taken to be the reciprocals of the squared standard error of slope S.E.$(m)$, the latter defined from Equation (4.20):

$$w_i = \frac{1}{[\text{S.E.}(m_i)]^2}. \tag{4.30}$$

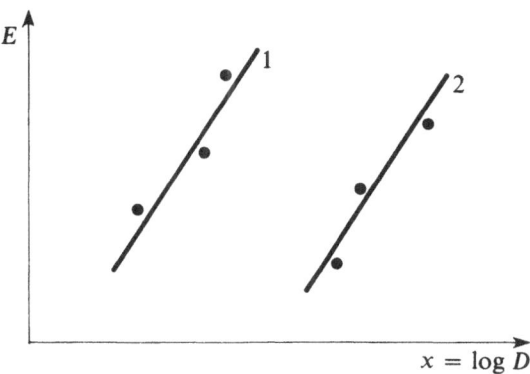

**Figure 4.13** Parallel line assays.

Using the average slope $m$, the equation of each line is written in the point-slope form. Using subscripts "1" and "2" for the means, we have for line 1

$$\hat{y} = \bar{y}_1 + m(x - \bar{x}_1), \tag{4.31}$$

and for line 2

$$\hat{y} = \bar{y}_2 + m(x - \bar{x}_2). \tag{4.32}$$

*Example.* Analgesia was tested in rats as a function of increasing doses of morphine sulfate administered subcutaneously. The dose–response curve is shown in Figure 4.14 (curve 1—broken). This same experiment was repeated

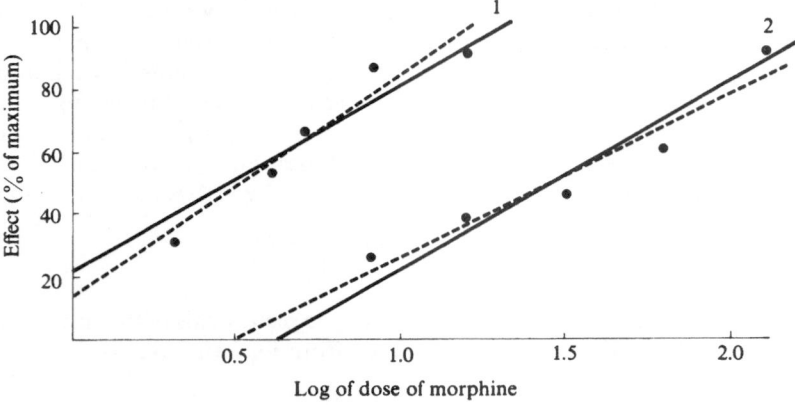

**Figure 4.14** The analgesic effect of morphine in rate is plotted against log dose (curve 1—broken). The antagonism produced by naloxone (0.05 mg/kg) is demonstrated by the shift of the curve to the right (curve 2—broken). The curves are redrawn as parallel lines (solid curves 1 and 2) in accord with the theory of competitive antagonism.

in the presence of a fixed dose of the antagonist naloxone, and the dose–response curve is shown in the figure (curve 2—broken). According to the theory of competitive antagonism, these curves should be parallel (see p. 61). The regression lines for each yielded the following statistics:

| Curve (1) | Curve (2) |
|---|---|
| $\bar{x} = 0.741$ | $\bar{x} = 1.51$ |
| $\bar{y} = 66.0$ | $\bar{y} = 52.8$ |
| $m = 72.4$ | $m = 52.9$ |
| $b = 12.3$ | $b = -26.8$ |
| S.E. $(m) = 11.7$ | S.E. $(m) = 8.17$ |
| $n = 5$ | $n = 5$ |

The weighting factor for curve (1) is $1/(11.7)^2 = 0.0073$, whereas that for curve (2) is $1/(8.17)^2 = 0.015$. The average slope is, from Equation (4.29),

$$m = \frac{(0.0073)(72.4) + (0.015)(52.9)}{0.0073 + 0.015}$$

$$= 59.3.$$

The equations of the parallel lines are $\hat{y} - 66 = 59.3(x - 0.741)$ and $\hat{y} - 52.8 = 59.3(x - 1.51)$. These are shown (solid) in Figure 4.14.

## Quantal Dose–Response Relation

Thus far we have discussed the *graded* dose–response curve, that is, the relation between the tissue (or species) response to increasing drug concentrations. We now discuss the quantal or "all-or-none" response to drug concentration. Suppose, for example, that we want to know how much of a hypnotic drug will produce hypnosis in rats. We would study a large number of rats, say 100, determining for each rat the smallest dose of drug that will produce sleep. Although there are different levels of sleep, we could define some particular end point, for example, failure to respond to a measured amount of pressure on the tail. In this test, therefore, there is just *one response*; either the rat is asleep or he is not, according to our chosen end point. Hence, the term "quantal." We could plot the histogram for the number, or percent, of rats that show the response for concentrations between 1 and 2 mg/kg, between 2 and 3 mg/kg, etc. Figure 4.15 shows a histogram of this type. An alternate way of representing these data is shown in Figure 4.16.

In Figure 4.16 the *cumulative distribution* is plotted as a function of the dose. Thus, each ordinate represents the total percent of rats who experienced the

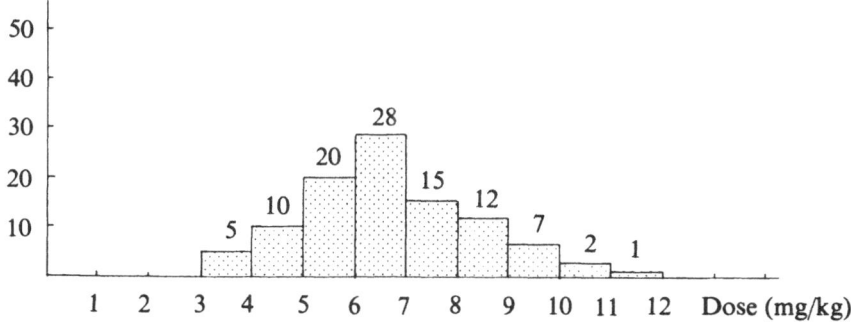

**Figure 4.15** Frequency distribution for hypnosis in rats.

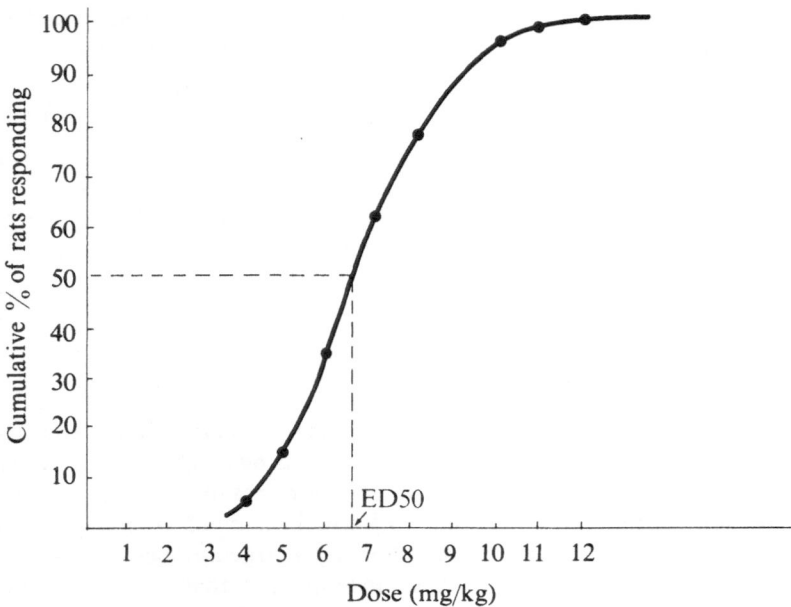

**Figure 4.16** The cumulative percent response, or quantal dose–response, curve.

effect with the dose (or some lower dose). The ordinate of this curve at any dose is numerically equal to the area under the histogram and to the left of the dose. This cumulative percent response relation is often called the "all-or-none," or quantal, dose–response relation.

The points in Figure 4.16 have been connected by a smooth curve. We are frequently interested in a single dose that tells us the potency of the drug. For this purpose we often state the *dose that produced the effect in 50% of the animals, the "ED50."* In the illustration the ED50 is 6.6 mg/kg.

In the illustration we chose hypnosis as the response. In fact, any other effect of the drug might have been chosen. For toxicological purposes we might have chosen some adverse effect, or even death. When death is the end point, *the dose that is lethal in 50% of the population is referred to as LD50.* Indeed, a drug that produces sleep can, in higher doses, be lethal. One may compare the LD50 and ED50 for the effect. A "safe" drug has a much larger LD50 than ED50. It is customary to use the ratio LD50/ED50 as an index of safety. This ratio is called the *therapeutic index.* When the therapeutic index of a drug is a small number, the drug must be used with extreme caution.

It is noteworthy that for many drugs the characteristic shape shown in the cumulative curve of Figure 4.16 is seen when the abscissa is expressed as log(concentration) rather than concentration.

## Probit Diagram

We have seen that the transformation $z = (x - \mu)/\sigma$ transforms any normal curve into a single, or standard, normal curve. An advantage of the transformation is that we can refer to one table which gives us the percentage area between two values of the standardized deviate $z$. The arithmetic mean of the distribution corresponds to $z = 0$ and, of course, the values of $z$ are both positive and negative since the variates are distributed around the mean.

Since our main interest is in the relation between the percentage area under the standard normal curve and the standardized normal deviate $z$ it is useful to display this relation. Thus, in Figure 4.17, as a vertical line is moved from left to right we determine *the area to the left of this line and plot it on the ordinate* as in Figure 4.18, producing a symmetrical sigmoid curve. In the diagrams $z = -1.5$ is shown. Reference to Table A.1 shows that the area corresponding to $z = 1.5$ is 0.4332. Since the total area to the left of $z = 0$ is 0.5, the shaded

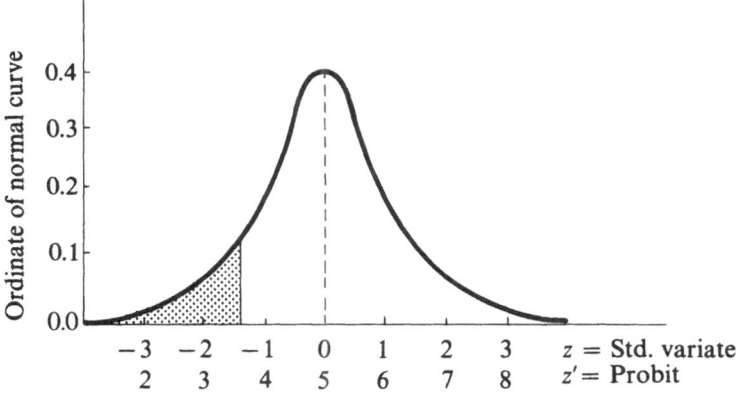

**Figure 4.17** Standardized normal distribution; shaded area is 6.68% of the total area and corresponds to $z = -1.5$.

area is 0.0668, or 6.68% of the total. Of course, $z = 0$ corresponds to 50% of the total area. In order to avoid negative values of the variate $z$ we can add some constant to each $z$. By convention we choose the constant 5, giving rise to a *probability unit* or *probit* $z'$. Hence $z' = z + 5$. The probit scale is shown on both Figures 4.17 and 4.18. The sigmoid curve of Figure 4.18 provides us with a correspondence between percentages of the total area under the standard normal curve and value of the probit. A table of probits is given in the appendix (Table A.3). More extensive tables of probits exist. We have constructed Table A.3 (as a convenience) by using Table A.1 (the area under the standard normal curve) and the definition $z' = z + 5$ in order to get the correspondence between any area and the probit.

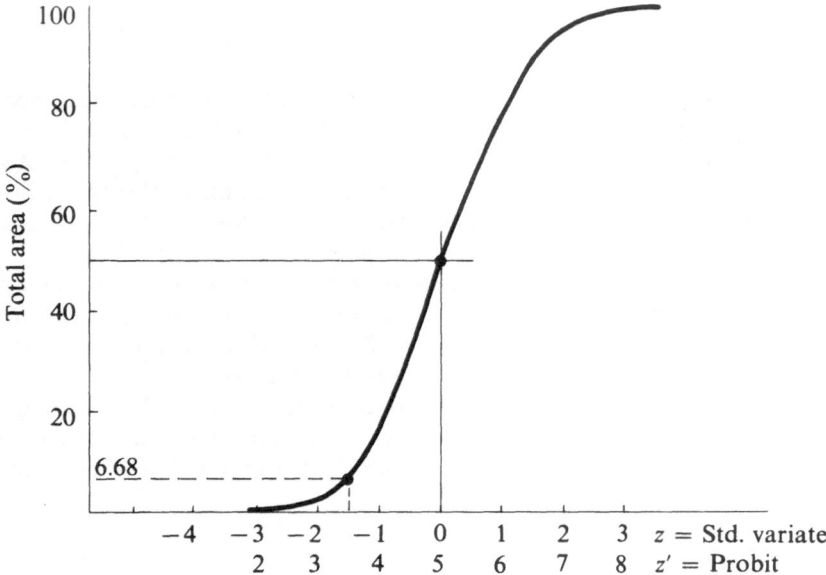

**Figure 4.18** Cumulative normal distribution. The variate $z = -1.5$ (shown) corresponds to probit $z' = 3.5$.

Suppose we were to plot the quantal dose–response curve of Figure 4.16 in a different way; instead of plotting the cumulative percentage of rats responding to a particular dose of drug, we plot instead the probit on the ordinate. The ordinate, then, is calibrated in units of the standard variate. For example, the 50 % value of area, representing a drug response in 50 % of the rats, corresponds to a probit of 5 for a dose of 6.6 mg/kg. The other points of the dose–response curve are listed in Table 4.1, from which the probit plot of Figure 4.19 results.

It is seen that the curve of Figure 4.19 is very nearly linear ($r = 0.99$). *A probit plot that is linear tells us that the distribution is normal.* Since departures from normality are not easily seen in the quantal dose–response curves, the probit plot is a convenient indicator that the distribution is normal. In many cases the probit plot of drug responses with concentration on the abscissa may not be

**Table 4.1**
The conversion of percent to probits for the dose–response curve of Figure 4.16

| Concentration | 4 | 5 | 6 | 7 | 8 | 9 | 10 | 11 | 12 |
|---|---|---|---|---|---|---|---|---|---|
| Cumulative % | 5 | 15 | 35 | 63 | 78 | 90 | 97 | 99 | 100 |
| Probit | 3.35 | 3.96 | 4.61 | 5.33 | 5.77 | 6.28 | 6.88 | 7.33 | 8.72[a] |

[a] Actually, 8.72 corresponds to 99.99 %.

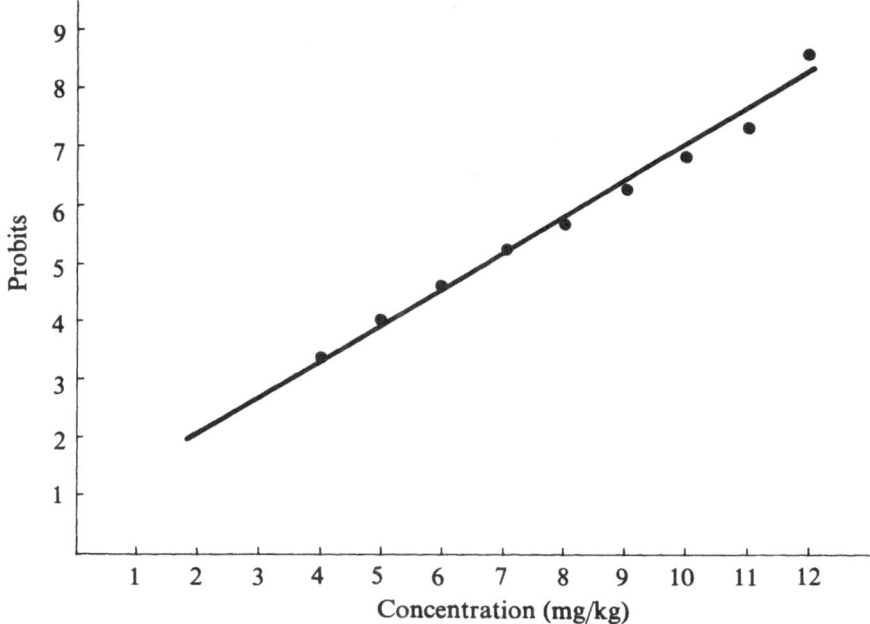

**Figure 4.19** Probit plot of Figure 4.16.

linear. In such cases, one should try plotting probits against the *logarithm of the concentration.* A linear probit plot in these cases tells us that the distribution is *lognormally distributed.*

Probit analysis, though very useful in estimating mean effective doses from quantal assays, requires a good deal of analysis. Prior to the widespread use of electronic computers the work was rather tedious. Consequently, certain simplifications in the method were introduced, the best known being that of Litchfield and Wilcoxon in 1949.[3] This system makes use of nomograms for determining the ED50, and it can also be used for determining a potency ratio, including a test for parallelism. Although it is still worthwhile for illustration, the general availability of computers in most schools and laboratories has reduced the importance of such "time-saving" methods. Many important statistical methods, including the principles of biological assay, and many experimental designs, are discussed in Finney's well-known book.

## References

1. Ariëns, E. J., Simonis, A. M., and Van Rossum: In *Molecular Pharmacology*, Vol. I. (E. J. Ariëns, ed.) New York, Academic Press, 1964, p. 144.
2. Gaddum, J. H.: Pharmacol. Rev., 5:87, 1953.

3. Litchfield, J. T., and Wilcoxon, F.: J. Pharmacol., *95*:99, 1949.
4. Perry, W. L. M.: Med. Research Council Spec. Rep. Ser., *270*:1, 1950.
5. Data supplied by Robert Raffa, Dept. of Pharmacology, Temple University School of Medicine, Philadelphia, Pa.
6. van Maanen, E. F.: J. Pharmacol. Exp. Ther., *99*:255, 1950.

## Additional Readings

Alder, H. L., and Roessler, E. B. *Introduction to Probability and Statistics*, 6th ed. San Francisco, W. H. Freeman, 1977.

Bliss, C. I. *Statistics in Biology I*, New York, McGraw-Hill, 1967.

Bourke, G. J., and McGilvray, J. *Interpretation and Uses of Medical Statistics*, 2nd ed. Oxford, Blackwell Scientific Publishers, 1975.

Dixon, W. J., and Massey, F. J. *Introduction to Statistical Analysis*, 3rd ed. New York, McGraw-Hill, 1969.

Draper, R. N., and Smith, H. *Applied Regression Analysis*. New York, John Wiley, 1966.

Dunn, O. J. *Basic Statistics: A Primer for the Biomedical Sciences*. New York, John Wiley, 1964.

Finney, D. J. *Experimental Design and Its Statistical Basis*. Chicago, University of Chicago Press, 1974.

Freund, J. E. *Statistics—A First Course*, 2nd ed. Englewood Cliffs, N.J.: Prentice-Hall, 1976.

Remington, R. D., and Schork, M. A. *Statistics with Applications to the Biological and Health Sciences*. Englewood Cliffs, N.J.: Prentice-Hall, 1970.

Tatsuoka, M. M. *Multivariate Analysis*. New York, John Wiley, 1971.

# Drug Binding and Drug Effect

## Chapter 5

### Receptor Interaction and Effect

Drugs that bind readily to a tissue may differ markedly in their ability to produce an effect. In other words, they differ in efficacy or in intrinsic activity. We do not know the reason for these differences; in fact, we do not know very much about the sequence of events between binding and effect. A reasonable explanation would seem to be access to the receptor. Clearly, if the drug molecule cannot arrive at the receptor, then no effect is possible. However, even when access to the receptor is not limited, the effect may not temporally follow the binding. For example, if acetylcholine is administered to a tissue, the effect can rise to a peak and then fall to some lower level, even though the concentration at the receptor is still apparently rising. As a specific example, we mention the work of Lullman and Ziegler,[33] who studied the time course of uptake of carbachol by the guinea pig atria and the time course of the effect, decreased contractile force. The time courses of effect and concentration were very different. The effect reached its final value in 2–3 min, whereas the uptake was still in progress even after 30 min. These are just two examples, but there are numerous others which suggest a temporal dependence in the concentration–effect relationship. Thus, access to the receptors is not a general explanation for differences in the efficacy. Furthermore, binding to the tissue may bear no relation to a drug's ability to produce an effect.

A view that is gaining in popularity is that the activation of a receptor by a drug may be a *quantal* rather than a graded transition. The rate theory of Paton (see p. 81) is one example of a quantal theory. In this theory the efficacy of a drug is related to its rate of turnover and is, therefore, related to the dissociation constant of the drug–receptor complex. Koshland[29] expanded on the rate theory, meshing it with the view that the receptor is elastic, and that it is the change in the receptor's tertiary structure that causes the effect. Thus, if drug–receptor binding results in such a conformational change that the drug binds less strongly and dissociates more easily, then the drug is an agonist. If, however, binding does not result in a change in configuration, the binding is stable and an antagonist rather than an agonist is involved. Efficacy, then, becomes a measure of the probability that a drug will result in an occupied receptor having the "active" conformation.

Allosteric theory is a quantal theory. The receptor exists in an active (R) form and in an inactive (T) form. The microscopic dissociation constants for binding molecule A to R and to T are $K_{AR}$ and $K_{AT}$, respectively. According to this view an antagonist acts competitively if it reacts with the same site as the agonist but has a relatively higher affinity for the T form than for the R form. Efficacy in this model is given by $(K_{AT}/K_{AR} - 1)$ and, for a strong agonist, $K_{AT}/K_{AR} \gg 1$, meaning high affinity for the R form. The allosteric model is an alternative to the occupation theory model in the analysis of pharmacological experiments.

Pharmacological data have not provided definitive evidence favoring any one of these models over the others, so that the question of mechanism remains unresolved.

> Working with human serum esterase which contains two receptor sites for morphine and related drugs, Gero[16] proposed the hypothesis that efficacy in this system may be related to distortion of the receptor. In this experimental system one of the drug–receptor sites accelerates the enzymatic hydrolysis of procain when the receptor is occupied; the effect, then, is the rate of hydrolysis, and the efficacy is measured from the *rate constant* of hydrolysis. The drugs of the series that had efficacy were those that forced the receptor to conform to the drug. Those that attached strainlessly were without effect.

## Binding Constants and Dissociation Constants

The attractive force between a drug molecule and its receptor is the resultant of forces due to several bond types. Probably the primary force is electrostatic attraction between the drug molecule and the receptor. The specificity and duration of drug action require, however, that the primary electrostatic action be reinforced by concomitant forces such as those due to hydrogen bonding and van der Waals attraction. Although some drug molecules form covalent bonds with their receptors, this type of strong bond is the exception rather than the rule. The complex resulting from the covalent binding of a drug with a receptor is essentially irreversible. Generally, covalent bonds are associated with toxic rather than pharmacological actions of drugs.

The determination of drug–receptor dissociation constants, as discussed in Chapter 3, uses *pharmacological* methods, that is, each method uses measurements of the *effect* produced by either a single drug or a combination of drugs. Three methods were presented for agonist drugs (see pp. 67–79) and one for antagonist drugs (see p. 61). In most cases these procedures are used on cellularly intact tissues in which a response such as muscle contraction or membrane electrical depolarization is measured. Thus, when the term "receptor" is used in the pharmacological literature, it refers to that (generally unknown) molecular constituent of the cell with which an active drug reacts to produce a *response*. The receptor is, therefore, something more than a binding site, a fact that has already been emphasized.

In an attempt to identify and quantify receptors by direct chemical or physical methods, several laboratories have worked with radioactive ligands of very high activity. These substances are used in homogenates or in membrane fractions of the tissue that is presumed to contain the receptor being studied. The advances in the procedures for fractionation, isolation, and purification of these sub-cellular constituents, and their high affinity for the labeled substance hold great promise for the identification of receptors. Of central importance in this identification of binding sites as receptors is the agreement in the values of drug–receptor dissociation constants determined by both radioligand binding methods and standard pharmacological methods. Furchgott,[15] who has developed and used pharmacological methods for determining dissociation constants, cautions "the investigator who claims to be studying a specific type of receptor with the radioligand procedure must validate his claim by showing good correlation between the values of the affinities of a series of antagonists and agonists for the specific sites to which the radioligand binds, and the values of affinities of the same series of agonists and antagonists for a specific receptor as derived from the results of appropriate pharmacological testing."

In order to compare dissociation constants determined by radioligand-binding procedures with those obtained by the pharmacological methods of Chapter 3, a substance having high affinity for the tissue is labeled with a radioactive agent such as tritium. The drug under study is then administered, thus reducing the binding of the radioligand. *If the concentration of radioligand is well below its own apparent K, then the dissociation constant of the drug is equal to the concentration of drug required to reduce binding of the radioligand by 50%.* This result follows from application of simple competitive theory as shown at the end of this section.

**Table 5.1**

Muscarinic receptors: Comparison of dissociation constants determined by radioligand-binding procedure and pharmacological procedures[a]

| Drug | $ID_{50}$ against binding of [$^3$H]QNB | $K_D$ estimated in pharmacological studies |
|---|---|---|
| Antagonists | | |
| Scopolamine | $2-3 \times 10^{-10}$ | $3 \times 10^{-10}$ |
| Atropine | $2-4 \times 10^{-9}$ | $1 \times 10^{-9}$ |
| Agonists | | |
| Acetylcholine | $2-4 \times 10^{-6}$ | $1.1 \times 10^{-6}$ |
| | | $2.4 \times 10^{-6}$ |
| Carbachol | $2-3 \times 10^{-5}$ | $1.2 \times 10^{-5}$ |
| Methacholine | $2-3 \times 10^{-6}$ | $3.9 \times 10^{-6}$ |
| Pilocarpine | $7-9 \times 10^{-7}$ | $3.3 \times 10^{-6}$ |
| | | $4.4 \times 10^{-6}$ |

[a] All values in moles per liter. From Furchgott.[15]

When comparisons were made using a membrane preparation from guinea pig intestinal smooth muscle, a group of muscarinic agents showed good agreement in the values of $K$ determined by both methods. The labeled agent in these experiments was [$^3$H]quinuclidinyl benzilate, or [$^3$H]QNB. Furchgott[15] has summarized the data, shown in Table 5.1.

Similarly, when dissociation constants of α-adrenergic agents were compared by Furchgott, the agreement was also good, as seen in Table 5.2. In these experiments the radioligand was [$^3$H]dihydroergocryptine, and the preparation was the membrane fraction of rabbit uterine smooth muscle. The pharmacological procedure used rabbit aortic smooth muscle. Tsai and Lefkowitz[60] used this same labeled α-adrenergic agent in their study on canine aortic receptors. Based on their results it was suggested that the binding sites of [$^3$H]dihydroergocryptine are the same as the α-adrenergic receptors.

Work with labeled compounds as a means of locating drug receptors is proceeding at a rapid pace for a variety of different receptors. Kebabian and Calne,[28] in their review of dopamine, discuss the progress with this methodology in locating dopaminergic receptors, while Hulme et al.[25] have studied brain muscarinic receptors, Mohler and Okada,[38] benzodiazepine receptors, and Akera,[1] a possible digitalis receptor. Giachetti and Shore[18] in their review of the reserpine receptor discuss the progress made in the identification of this receptor with tritiated reserpine.

In recent years there has been much work done with stereospecific binding of opiates using particulate tissue preparations from animal or human brain. Simon and Hiller[50,51] nicely summarize the progress made in the study of

**Table 5.2**

$\alpha$-Adrenergic receptors: Comparison of dissociation constants determined by radioligand-binding procedure and pharmacological procedures[a]

| Drug | Radioligand binding | Pharmacological studies |
|------|---------|---------|
| Antagonists | | |
| Phentolamine | 0.015 | 0.015 |
| Dihydroergotamine | 0.015 | 0.005 |
| Propranolol | 27 | 6.8 |
| Agonists | | |
| ( − )-Norepinephrine | 0.65 | 0.24 |
| ( − )-Epinephrine | 0.23 | 0.21 |
| ( − )-Phenylephrine | 3.5 | 1.1 |
| $\alpha$-Methyl-NE | 2.3 ( ± ) | 2.8 ( − ) |
| ( ± )-$\alpha$-Ethyl-NE | 100 | 74 |
| Dopamine | 21 | 64 |

[a] Values represent dissociation constants ($K_D$) in micromoles per liter. From Furchgott.[15]

the opiate "receptor." A comparison of the dissociation constants of various opiates determined by the radiolabeled procedure and standard pharmacological procedures has not been accomplished as of the time of this writing. The reason is that values of $K$ for opiates have not been determined by pharmacological methods. However, there is a good correlation between the pharmacological potency of a large number of opiates and their affinity for binding to brain tissue. The reader is urged to consult the several excellent sources for further information on this exciting area of narcotic research.[19,23,32,43,53,59]

A radiolabeled compound with dissociation constant $K_A$ is given in a concentration $A$ which is much less than $K_A$. The fractional binding is, from Equation (3.4), $A/(A + K_A)$. It is desired to determine the dissociation constant $K_B$ of a drug (unlabeled) which has affinity for the same binding site as that of the labeled compound. Equation (3.20) for competitive antagonism is applicable, that is, the fraction of receptor bound by the labeled agent is reduced to

$$\frac{A}{A + K_A(1 + B/K_B)}$$

where $B$ is the drug concentration. We wish to determine the concentration of $B$ which reduces the binding of the labeled agent by 50%. Hence

$$\frac{A}{A + K_A(1 + B/K_B)} = \frac{1}{2} \cdot \frac{A}{A + K_A}.$$

Rearrangement yields $(B/K_B - 1) = A/K_A$. Since $A \ll K_A$, the right-hand side $\approx 0$ and $B = K_B$. Thus, this concentration $B$, called $ID_{50}$, is numerically equal to the dissociation constant of the drug.

## Desensitization

In many pharmacological preparations it is found that the response to a given concentration of drug is diminished (or abolished) after prior exposure to the same or to a different drug. For example, if an isolated preparation of guinea pig ileum is given a large dose of acetylcholine, the tissue will be temporarily insensitive to a subsequent dose of *either* acetylcholine or histamine.[7] In the fowl rectal cecum the response to histamine is abolished by a prior soaking of the tissue in histamine, but the response to other drugs such as acetylcholine and epinephrine is only slightly diminished.[5] The diminution in response in either case is called *desensitization*, and it may be either drug-specific, as in the fowl cecum, or non-drug-specific, as in the guinea pig ileum. Obviously, in those preparations that exhibit desensitization the experimental procedure for getting replicable dose–response data is complicated. If such a preparation is dosed cumulatively, the drug washed out, and the preparation dosed again, the dose–response curves will not be the same. An example using an adrenergic preparation is given in Figure 5.1. Curve 1 represents isometric tension in isolated rabbit aorta as a function of increasing concentrations of norepinephrine. Curve 2 represents a repetition of the experiment 30 min after the completion of a wash-out of the drug. Curve 2 is displaced to the right over an appreciable range of effects but attains the same maximum in this case. Thus potency is decreased and efficacy remains constant. Several theoretical models have been proposed for the phenomenon of desensitization, and some of these are discussed subsequently. For now, we continue to examine the consequences of desensitization on the dose–response curve.

MacNab[37] studied specific and nonspecific desensitization on the isolated rabbit aortic strip. He considered the effects of time for recovery and the degree of passive tension (preloading) on the tissue response. When norepinephrine was the stimulating drug, it was found that the recovery of sensitivity, indicated by the left-to-right position of the curve, after a maximal dose of drug depends on the amount of passive tension. With large tensions (10-g preload) the recovery of sensitivity did not occur even after 5 hr. When the preload was 2 g or less, restoration of sensitivity did occur after approximately 2 hr; i.e., the potency was restored. The maximum response ($E_{max}$) was also found to be dependent upon the preload. With 10 g there was just a slight decrease in $E_{max}$ (2%) and this level was constant over time (although the potency remained depressed). For the 2-g preload the maximum response actually increased by about 15%, 3 hr after the initial dosing.

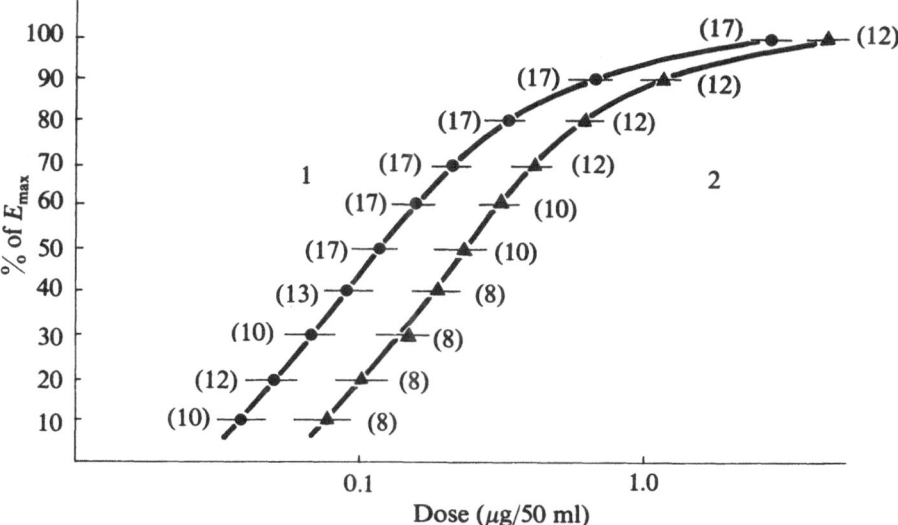

**Figure 5.1** Desensitization to norepinephrine in strips of rabbit thoracic aorta. Curve 1 (●) is the first dose–response curve. Curve 2 (▲) was obtained 30 min later on the same prepara- tion and was preceded by several washes after which the tension (isometric) returned to zero. The numbers in parentheses refer to the number of strips used at each level of response. The plotted points represent mean concentrations, and the horizontal lines indicate the standard error of the mean. Abscissa: micrograms of drug in a 50 ml bath. (From MacNab.[37])

Desensitization is obviously a complicating factor in experiments in which antagonist drugs are used, such as in the determination of dissociation constants (see Chap. 3). In such experiments the degree of shift of the curve due to de- sensitization must be separated from that attributable to the antagonist. One way of getting around this complication is to avoid redosing on the same tissue. Thus, one must determine a *mean* concentration–response curve derived from first exposures of a sample of tissues in the absence of the antagonist. In the same way, a mean concentration–response curve for first exposure to the agonist must be determined in the presence of a fixed concentration of antagonist. Computa- tions are then made from the mean curves.

If the effect of the antagonist on the same preparation is to be accomplished, one must be certain that the recovery of agonist sensitivity is complete at the time the antagonist is administered. For example, in experiments on the isolated aortic strip previously described, sensitivity was restored after 2 hr, provided that the preload was 2 g. Hence, after 2 hr, dosing with agonist in the presence of antagonist could proceed. The shift in the curve is then attributable to the antagonist only. In any particular preparation the characteristics of desensitiza- tion and recovery should be determined prior to experimentation with the blocking drug.

One of the earliest models for desensitization was made by Del Castillo and Katz.[13] This model adheres to the theory of drug action that says that the response is a function of the number of receptors occupied by agonist molecules, but it adds a step to explain desensitization. If A is the agonist, R the receptor, and AR the drug–receptor complex,

$$A + R \underset{\text{fast}}{\rightleftharpoons} AR \underset{\text{slow}}{\rightleftharpoons} AR'.$$

The active complex AR slowly turns into an inactive form AR'. Desensitization results from the slow conversion to AR', and recovery from desensitization follows from slow reconversion of AR' to AR. Katz and Thesleff[27] made a more elaborate model, a cyclical model:

$$
\begin{array}{ccc}
A + R & \underset{\text{fast}}{\rightleftharpoons} & AR \\
\text{slow} \updownarrow & & \updownarrow \text{slow} \\
A + R' & \underset{\text{fast}}{\rightleftharpoons} & AR'
\end{array}
$$

Rang and Ritter[45] studied desensitization to cholinergic agents in chick and leech muscle. These results are compatible with the cyclic model, with the additional factor that certain drugs may have a preferential affinity for desensitized receptors.

Gero[17] used both models and the mass action law and formulated a theory in which the drug effect is a consequence of a distortion of the receptor brought about by interaction with the drug molecule. In this theory, desensitization (and drug dependence) follow as necessary consequences.

Waud[63] expresses skepticism about both receptor models, reasoning that the phenomena seen by Katz and Thesleff[27] could be explained by changes in events following receptor activation and adding that there is no reason to believe that desensitization is just one process. In particular, Waud views nonspecific desensitization as a form of "fatigue."


## Molecularity and Order

Up to this point we have considered the reaction between drug A and receptor R to follow the model $A + R \rightleftharpoons AR$; that is, one molecule of A combines with one molecule of R to form one molecule of AR. Suppose, however, that the drug–receptor reaction is

$$2A + R \rightleftharpoons A_2R.$$

In this case the *law of chemical equilibrium*, as formulated by Guldberg and Waage,[20] leads to

$$\frac{A^2 r}{X_e} = K \tag{5.1}$$

where $A, r,$ and $X_e$ are the equilibrium concentrations of drug, unbound receptor, and complex, respectively, and $K$ is the dissociation constant. It is useful to rearrange Equation (5.1) in order to express the concentration of complex $X_e$ in terms of the total receptor concentration $r_t$ and the drug concentration $A$. The concentration of A at equilibrium is assumed to be the same as the initial concentration (see Chap. 3). The equilibrium value of $r$, however, is the total minus the amount used to form the product:

$$r = r_t - X_e. \tag{5.2}$$

Substitution of Equation (5.2) into Equation (5.1) and rearrangement yield

$$X_e = \frac{A^2 r_t}{A^2 + K}. \tag{5.3}$$

The reader should compare Equation (5.3) with Equation (3.4). Since two molecules of drug react with one molecule of receptor, the drug concentration term is raised to the power 2. In general, if $n$ molecules of drug reacted with one molecule of receptor, the concentration term would have power $n$:

$$X_e = \frac{A^n r_t}{A^n + K}. \tag{5.4}$$

Since we can measure *effect* and not $X_e$, the binding function of Equation (5.4) is a theoretical construct. If it is *assumed* that the effect $E$ is directly proportional to $X_e$, Equation (5.4) leads to

$$E = \frac{E_{max} A^n}{A^n + K} \tag{5.5}$$

where $E_{max}$ is the maximal effect. Fitting (by least squares) actual concentration-effect data to Equation (5.5) in order to determine the best integral value of $n$ leads to a mechanistic interpretation of the concentration–effect data, namely, that $n$ molecules of drug combine with the receptor. Such interpretations have been criticized because the proportionality assumption is probably not generally applicable and, therefore, the shape of the concentration–effect curve is not helpful in revealing the concentration–occupancy relationship.[63]

Returning to the reaction $2A + R \rightleftharpoons A_2 R$, we have 3 molecules of reactants used to form the complex. This is an example of a *trimolecular* reaction; in other words, the *molecularity* is 3, whereas the usual model assumes a *bimolecular* reaction.

Figure 5.2 shows graphs of the concentration of drug–receptor complex against $A$ for each of the two situations, bimolecular and trimolecular. As mentioned above, one might compare the shape of individual dose–effect curves with each of these and, thus, postulate the molecularity of the drug–receptor reaction. It should be remembered, however, that, in general, the relation between the effect and the concentration of complex is not known.

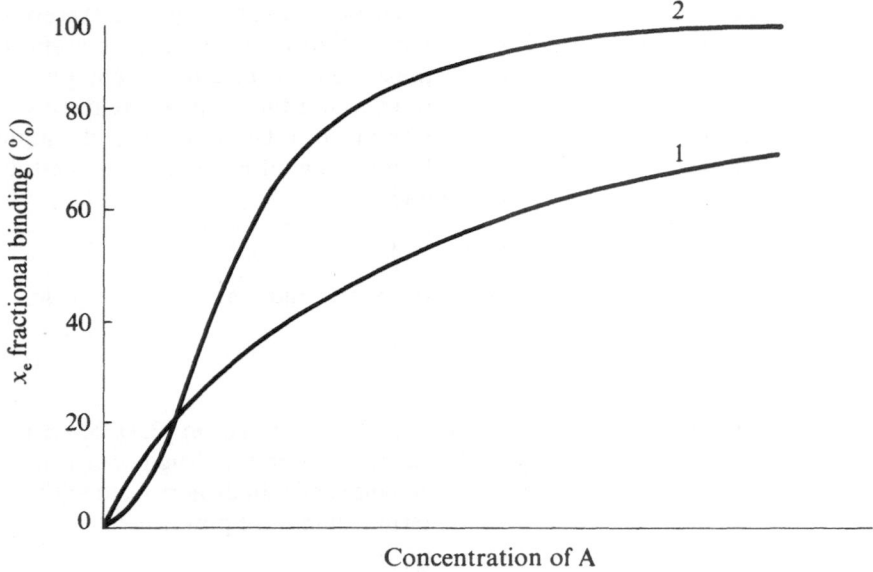

**Figure 5.2** Fraction of bound receptor against concentration: for bimolecular (1) and tri-molecular (2) reactions according to Equation (5.4).

Furthermore, even in *chemical* reactions in which the concentrations of reactants and products as functions of time are known, there is no necessary connection between the stoichiometry and the kinetic model (rate equation) which best fits the data.

Theoretical expressions for reaction rates as functions of concentrations are written as *differential equations*, that is, equations in which the rate of appearance or disappearance is expressed as a derivative. Thus, suppose in the reaction A + B → C + D the rate of disappearance of A, denoted $dC_A/dt$, is found to obey the rate equation

$$\frac{-dC_A}{dt} = KC_A{}^a \cdot C_B{}^b$$

where $C_B$ is the concentration of B at any time $t$ and $K$, $a$, and $b$ are constants. The *order* of the reaction is defined as the sum of the exponents, $a + b$. The order of a reaction need not be a whole number; it may be zero or a fraction. The reaction order is determined by integrating the rate equation and finding the values of $a$ and $b$ which best fit the experimental data. Sometimes even a simple unimolecular reaction will have a fractional order even though the stoichiometry might suggest order one. Examples of chemical reactions which emphasize the lack of connection between stoichiometry and order are given by Moore.*

A theoretical paper[57] examined the importance of molecularity and order on the determination of drug–receptor dissociation constants. We will give here only one example. Suppose that the reaction between drug and receptor is $2A + R \rightleftharpoons A_2R$. How does this reaction of higher molecularity affect the method for determining the dissociation constant discussed in Chapter 3 (p. 68)? In that method, a fraction $(1 - q)$ of the total receptor concentration is irreversibly inactivated, and equiactive agonist concentrations, $A$ and $A'$, before and after inactivation, are determined. Equation (3.24) applies to that case, yielding a straight line when $1/A$ is plotted against $1/A'$. In the trimolecular reaction under discussion the equation corresponding to Equation (3.24) is

$$\frac{1}{A^2} = \frac{1}{q} \cdot \frac{1}{A'^2} + \frac{1/q - 1}{K}. \tag{5.6}$$

Thus, the plot of $1/A$ against $1/A'$ is not a straight line in this case.

## Pharmacokinetic Considerations

In order for a drug to exert an effect in some target organ, the drug must be absorbed by the organ. A brief discussion of transfer between compartments is presented below. Detailed discussions are given in several books.[30,46,62]

For our purposes a compartment is a space into which a drug distributes; for example, blood may be considered a compartment, and brain, another compartment. It is assumed that the drug in any one part of a compartment can interchange rapidly with the drug in all other parts of the compartment; hence, we are not concerned about the transport of the substance within the compartment. If the drug is distributed slowly, we would have to postulate not one, but two or more compartments. In general, the distribution of the drug will not be uniform throughout the compartment; however, what is required of a compartment is that an increase or decrease of drug in any part will affect the entire compartment and result in a proportional increase or decrease in other parts of the compartment. Often we measure the concentration $C$ of a drug in some region of the compartment and "pretend" that the entire quantity $(Q)$ of the drug is at a uniform concentration equal to that of the region. The ratio $Q/C$ is then the *apparent volume of distribution V* with respect to the drug and the compartment.

Figure 5.3 illustrates in schematic form two compartments, labeled 1 and 2, separated by a thin membrane M. A quantity $Q_T$ of solute is introduced into compartment 1 and we follow the time course of this *closed* system as it approaches equilibrium without giving details about the mechanisms of transfer.

* See reference 20, p. 332.

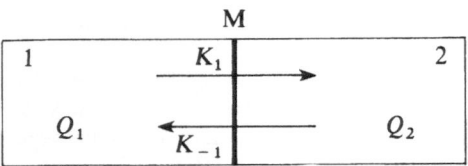

**Figure 5.3** A closed two-compartment system.

With certain qualifications, the model presented is applicable to a large class of real processes, both in vivo and in vitro. Actual transport across specific biological membranes is, however, often more complicated than this simple model depicts.[22,48]

It is assumed that the solute is uniformly distributed within each compartment and that there is a negligible quantity of solute within M. Then the rate of loss from compartment 1 is equal to the rate of gain of compartment 2. We denote the total quantity of solute by $Q_T$ and the instantaneous quantities of solute in compartments 1 and 2 by $Q_1$ and $Q_2$, respectively. Then the rate of change in compartment 1 is $dQ_1/dt$ and

$$\frac{dQ_1}{dt} = -K_1 Q_1 + K_{-1} Q_2. \tag{5.7}$$

Equation (5.7) states that the change in $Q_1$ is due to a loss proportional to $Q_1$ and a gain proportional to $Q_2$. The $K_1$ and $K_{-1}$ are rate constants, $K_1$ being the rate constant for passage from compartment 1 to compartment 2 and $K_{-1}$ for passage from compartment 2 to compartment 1. Since $Q_1 + Q_2 = Q_T$ (because the system is closed and we assume a negligible amount in the membrane), we may replace $Q_2$ by $Q_T - Q_1$ in Equation (5.7); hence,

$$\frac{dQ_1}{dt} = -K_1 Q_1 + K_{-1}(Q_T - Q_1)$$

or

$$\frac{dQ_1}{dt} = -(K_1 + K_{-1})Q_1 + K_{-1} Q_T. \tag{5.8}$$

The solution of Equation (5.8) gives the time course of $Q_1$. [Details of the solution of Equation (5.8) are given below for the interested reader.]

$$Q_1 = \frac{Q_T}{K_1 + K_{-1}} \{K_{-1} + K_1 \exp[-(K_1 + K_{-1})t]\}. \tag{5.9}$$

The quantity in compartment 2, $Q_2$, is most easily obtained from the difference $Q_2 = Q_T - Q_1$ which, after simplification, becomes

$$Q_2 = \frac{K_1 Q_T}{K_1 + K_{-1}} \{1 - \exp[-(K_1 + K_{-1})t]\}. \tag{5.10}$$

Graphs of $Q_1$ and $Q_2$ against time are given in Figure 5.4.

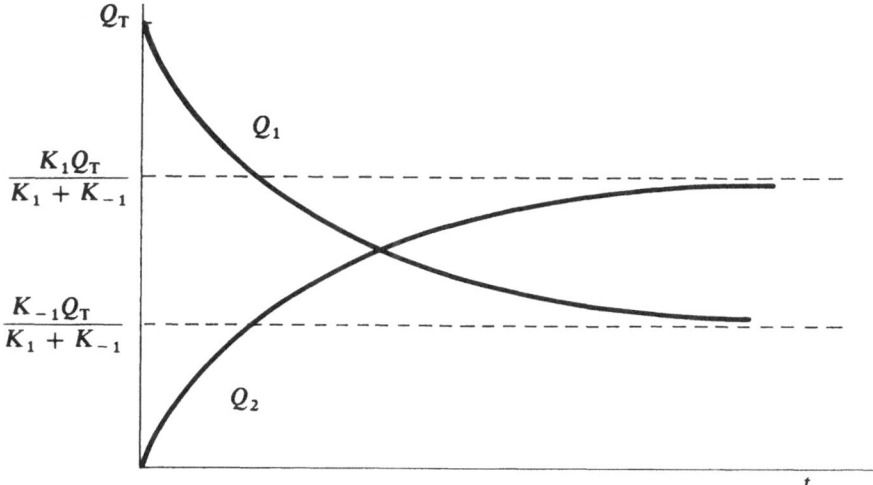

**Figure 5.4** Solution for the closed two-compartment model. In this illustration $K_1 > K_{-1}$.

The model previously discussed is applicable to a closed system; that is, a system in which the sum of the quantities $Q_1$ and $Q_2$ is instantaneously equal to the total drug $Q_T$ introduced into the system. When, however, there are pathways out of the system, the previous equations are not applicable. A common situation in pharmacology occurs when a drug is eliminated from one or both of the compartments as shown schematically in Figure 5.5. In the whole animal, compartment 1 is often the plasma and the elimination is due to metabolism and renal excretion. Metabolism, or transfer to a third compartment, or both, accounts for the pathway out of the system via compartment 2. The symbols $K_1'$ and $K_2'$ are rate constants for elimination from compartments 1 and 2, respectively. The general solution for this case is given, without derivation, below.

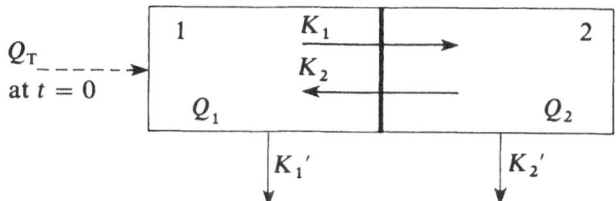

**Figure 5.5** An open two-compartment system.

Equation (5.8) is linear and of order 1. [See Equation (A.13) in Appendix C.] When put into *standard form* the equation becomes

$$dQ_1 + (K_1 + K_{-1})Q_1 \, dt = K_{-1}Q_T \, dt.$$

The integrating factor is $\exp[(K_1 + K_{-1})t]$. Hence,

$$Q_1 = \frac{\int \exp[(K_1 + K_{-1})t] \cdot K_{-1} \cdot Q_T \, dt}{\exp[(K_1 + K_{-1})t]} + \frac{C}{\exp[(K_1 + K_{-1})t]}$$

$$= \frac{K_{-1}Q_T}{(K_1 + K_{-1})} + \frac{C}{\exp[(K_1 + K_2)t]}. \tag{5.11}$$

At $t = 0$, $Q_1 = Q_T$; hence, solving for $C$ gives

$$C = Q_T\left(1 - \frac{K_{-1}}{K_1 + K_{-1}}\right).$$

Substitution into Equation (5.11) and simplification yields Equation (5.9).

$$Q_1 = \frac{Q_T}{K_1 + K_{-1}} \{K_{-1} + K_1 \exp[-(K_1 + K_{-1})t]\}.$$

For the open two-compartment system the total dose $Q_T$ is assumed to be entirely in compartment 1 at time $t = 0$. At a subsequent time $t$, the amount in compartment 1 will be denoted by $Q_1(t)$, and the amount in compartment 2 will be denoted by $Q_2(t)$. These amounts are given by

$$Q_1(t) = Q_T\left\{\left(\frac{\alpha - \beta + \gamma}{2\gamma}\right)\exp[-\tfrac{1}{2}(\alpha + \beta - \gamma)t]\right\}$$

$$+ Q_T\left\{\left(1 - \frac{\alpha - \beta + \gamma}{2\gamma}\right)\exp[-\tfrac{1}{2}(\alpha + \beta - \gamma)t]\right\} \tag{5.12}$$

and

$$Q_2(t) = Q_T\frac{K_1}{\gamma} \{\exp[-\tfrac{1}{2}(\alpha + \beta - \gamma)t] - \exp[-\tfrac{1}{2}(\alpha + \beta + \gamma)t]\} \tag{5.13}$$

where

$$\begin{aligned} \alpha &= K_1 + K_1' \\ \beta &= K_2 + K_2' \\ \gamma &= (\alpha - \beta)^2 + 4K_1K_2. \end{aligned} \tag{5.14}$$

## In Vivo Considerations

When experiments are conducted on intact animals, the dose–response data obtained, although useful for determining potency and effectiveness, are not easily applied to the determination of dissociation constants. There are two major reasons in addition to the kinds of theoretical objections to certain assumptions of the classical theory. First, the effect produced by a given dose of drug may not be a direct effect, that is, the effect may be due partly to some secondary action such as a reflex. This is the case, for example, when blood pressure is determined as a function of increasing doses of a vascoconstricting drug. As the pressure increases with increasing doses, the baroreceptors in the carotid sinus and the aortic arch are stimulated, causing a reflex sympathetic inhibition which partly masks the direct action. Hence, a dose–response curve for an agonist drug has limited usefulness in such cases. A pair of curves, however, one for agonist alone and the other for agonist plus antagonist, can be useful for determining the dissociation constant of the antagonist, provided we assume that equal effects mean equal agonist–receptor binding (see Chap. 3).

The second point to be considered when experimenting with an intact organism is the tissue concentration of drug and its relation to the administered dose. From the previous section we know that the tissue concentration depends on the dose and on the time. From the integrated solution of the *theoretical model it is readily seen that the peak tissue concentration is proportional to the dose*, as shown in Figure 5.6. In the figure we show a graph, derived from Equation (5.13), for two different administered doses, $Q_{T1}$ and $Q_{T2} = 2Q_{T1}$. Shown are the tissue concentrations $C_1$ and $C_2$, as functions of time, corresponding to each of the administered doses.

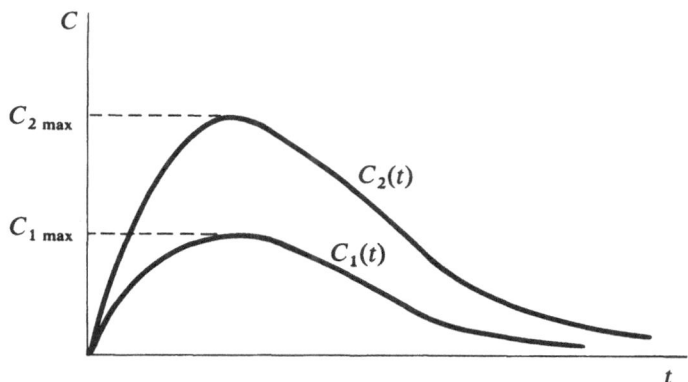

**Figure 5.6** Illustration of tissue concentrations. The ratio $C_{2\,max}/C_{1\,max}$ equals the ratio of administered doses $Q_{T2}/Q_{T1}$. In this illustration the ratio is 2.

The proportionality between administered dose and peak tissue concentration has been the basis for the determination of dissociation constants of antagonist agents from experiments conducted in vivo. Most noteworthy are the experiments aimed at determining the $K_B$, or $pA_2$ $(= -\log K_B)$, of opiate antagonists such as naloxone using various narcotic analgesics as agonists.[55,56,58] In these experiments the dosage schedule is such that at the time of measurement of effect, both the agonist (e.g., morphine) and the antagonist are at their respective maximum concentrations, $C_{A\,max}$ and $C_{B\,max}$. The Schild method (see Chap. 3) requires the use of these tissue concentrations in Equation (3.13). However, since proportionality between administered doses and maximum

**Table 5.3**

Examples of in vivo $pA_2$ values for naloxone and nalorphine in combination with various strong analgesics[a]

| Test/reference | Agonist/antagonist | $pA_2$(95%, C.L.'s) | Slope $\pm$ S.E. |
|---|---|---|---|
| Benzoquinone-induced | Methadone/naloxone | 6.98(6.71–7.24) | −0.79 ± 0.09 |
| stretching in mice[52] | Morphine/naloxone | 7.08(6.86–7.29) | −0.83 ± 0.03 |
| | Pentazocine/naloxone | 6.20(6.01–6.40) | −1.74 ± 0.05 |
| Mouse hot plate test[21] | Morphine/naloxone | 7.27(7.02–7.52) | −1.08 |
| Mouse tail flick test[21] | Morphine/naloxone | 7.10(7.10–7.10) | −1.20 |
| Hyperthermia in mice[35] | Morphine/naloxone | 6.57(6.44–6.70) | −1.35 ± 0.01 |
| Respiratory depression in mice[35] | Morphine/naloxone | 7.35(7.30–7.40) | −1.18 ± 0.02 |
| Rat tail flick test [66] | Morphine/ naloxone (intrathecally) | 8.20 | −1.1 |
| Rat hot plate test[66] | Morphine/ naloxone (intrathecally) | 8.05 | −1.1 |
| Rat tail compression test[10] | Morphine/naloxone | 8.1(7.7–8.5) | Constrained to unity |
| | Ethylketocyclazocine/ naloxone | 8.1(7.7–8.6) | Constrained to unity |

[a] From Tallarida et al.[56] with permission of Life Sci.

tissue concentrations is assumed, the calculation of $pA_2$ in vivo is accomplished by substitution of the administered dose. Hence, the in vivo $pA_2$ values are numbers which have associated with them the route of administration. It is reasoned that, to the extent that differences in $K$ values or $pA_2$'s permit a quantitative separation of receptors, these values, when determined in vivo, have this same fundamental usefulness. Table 5.3 is a partial list of $pA_2$ values determined from experiments on intact animals.* (See reference 56.)

The $pA_2$ is a measure of the affinity of an antagonist for the receptor. It is quite reasonable, therefore, to expect that this measure might be useful in revealing the mechanism of tolerance to narcotics†; in other words, is tolerance due to a decreased affinity for the narcotic receptor? An answer to this question based on values of $pA_2$ in vivo does not exist presently, largely because a measure of in vivo $pA_2$ with the degree of precision needed to shed light on this question has not been made.

An alternate approach has been the determination of the binding of various narcotics to brain tissue and the displacement of the narcotic with antagonists. Experiments of this type have produced conflicting results. Shen and Way[49] reported a dramatic drop in morphine concentration in the brain when naloxone

* The slopes of the Schild plots are shown in column 4 of the table. Competitive theory requires a slope of −1 in such plots (see also Chap. 3).

† See also the discussion of desensitization in Chapter 5.

was given to dependent animals (mice). No such change could be found by Dum et al.[14] in either naive or morphine-tolerant mice, even in response to a large naloxone dose. They suggested that the portion of the receptor-bound opiate in relation to the total amount bound to brain might be too low to detect. Höllt et al.[24] did find, however, that naloxone could displace brain levels of more potent narcotics (such as etorphine) with high affinity, this in contrast to opiates of lower affinity. Interestingly, the longitudinal muscle-myenteric plexus preparation from the guinea pig (see also Chap. 6) is frequently used to assess morphine action and morphine binding as correlates of the in vivo actions of the narcotic. Cox[11] reported that animals pretreated with morphine and then studied in vitro using this preparation showed a reduction in morphine sensitivity, but this reduction was not associated with alterations in opiate receptor binding. These results provide some insight into the limitations of both binding and $pA_2$ studies in relation to answering certain questions regarding drug action. Refinements of methodology may yet provide answers.

The use of in vivo $pA_2$ values for answering other questions about drug action continues to be widespread. For example, Szekely et al.[54] used in vivo $pA_2$ values obtained for naloxone against morphine, $\beta$-endorphin, and a synthetic enkephalin analog in order to learn whether the receptor mediating the analgesic response for each was the same. They concluded that in mice the same receptor exists for both morphine and the opioid peptides, but in rats there may be different receptors. Tulunay[61] measured $pA_2$'s for naloxone with morphine and butorphanol in the rat, using hyperthermia as the effect. He found significant differences in the $pA_2$ values obtained from each drug pair and suggested, therefore, that "narcotic and narcotic antagonist analgesics appear to interact with receptors in different manners." McGilliard and Takemori[36] obtained $pA_2$ values for naloxone-morphine using two narcotic effects, analgesia and respiratory depression, in both naive and morphine pretreated mice. They interpreted their measured differences in $pA_2$ values to mean that narcotic-induced respiratory depression and analgesia are mediated through different morphine receptors. On the other hand, Cowan et al.[10] attempted to differentiate the two postulated morphine receptors ($\mu$ and $\kappa$)[34] by determining the in vivo $pA_2$ for naloxone against narcotic analgesics presumed to be specific for each receptor type. They found differences in the $pA_2$ values, but the wide 95% confidence limits precluded their making a firm conclusion about whether one or two receptors were involved, thus emphasizing the importance of the precision of this measure when making conclusions about receptors.

## Protein Binding

Many drugs accumulate in body compartments that are unrelated to their locus of action. These compartments act as reservoirs or depots for the drug and thus affect the distribution of the drug throughout the organism; in particular, binding of this kind can limit the biophase concentration of a drug. Notable among these binding sites are the *plasma proteins*, most importantly, plasma *albumin*. The degree of binding and the strength of the bond will vary from one drug to another. Because it limits the transport to the receptor, significant binding to plasma proteins can thus have a profound effect on the pharmacological response and, consequently, on the dose–response relation. All excretory pathways may be affected by protein binding. For illustrating the principles, however, it is sufficient to discuss the kidney, since it is the most important organ for excreting drugs and drug metabolites, and, in particular, renal glomerular filtration.

Only the free drug in plasma water, i.e., that which is *not bound* to plasma proteins or other tissue, can be filtered by the renal glomerular capillaries.* Thus, if a drug is highly bound, its clearance (expressed as volume of plasma water per unit time) is low. Now the first-order rate constant $k$ for elimination (discussed in Chap. 2) is related to the clearance $Cl$ and the apparent volume of distribution $V_d$ according to

$$k = \frac{Cl}{V_d}. \tag{5.15}$$

The value of $k$, in turn, is related to the half-life $t_{1/2}$ according to Equation (2.24): $k = \ln 2/t_{1/2}$; thus

$$t_{1/2} = (\ln 2)\frac{V_d}{Cl}. \tag{5.16}$$

Equation (5.16) gives a general relationship between half-life, clearance, and volume of distribution. Obviously, the apparent volume of distribution and the clearance are not independent of each other. In fact, both are parameters whose values are related to a *model*; nevertheless, the relation expressed by Equation (5.16), derived heuristically, expresses a rather general rule, namely, the larger the value of $V_d$, the longer is the half-life. Thus, substances that are highly bound to plasma proteins, thereby giving a large apparent volume of distribution (which may greatly exceed actual body water volume), will have long half-lives. Put differently, Equation (5.16) expresses the common sense fact that the smaller the clearance, the greater the half-life.

The interaction between a drug D and the protein P may be viewed as a simple reversible reaction

$$D + P \rightleftharpoons DP$$

and, hence, describable in terms of the mass action law, leading to the *equilibrium* expression

$$K = \frac{(D)(P)}{(DP)}, \tag{5.17}$$

---

* Renal tubular secretion of bound agents does occur.

where $(D)$ is the concentration of free drug, $(P)$ is the free protein concentration, and $(DP)$ the concentration of occupied binding sites, all at equilibrium. The total protein concentration $(P)_t$ is the sum of $(P)$ and $(DP)$. Proceeding as in Chapter 3, we are led to

$$(DP) = \frac{(P)_t(D)}{(D) + K}.$$  (5.18)

The fraction of *drug bound* to protein, denoted by $r$, is

$$r = \frac{(DP)}{(D) + (DP)}.$$  (5.19)

From Equations (5.18) and (5.19) we get for the bound fraction

$$r = \frac{(P)_t}{(P)_t + (D) + K}.$$  (5.20)

Note that if $K$ is small (meaning a high binding affinity) the fraction $r$ will be large. Also, if $(D)$ is very large, the *fraction* of drug bound to protein decreases, as seen from Equation (5.20); however, the amount of binding becomes large, approaching $(P)_t$. In other words, there is high binding, but the drug concentration is so high that the fraction bound is small. We see, therefore, that knowledge of the bound fraction alone tells us little if we do not know the free drug concentration.

The preceding discussion which led to Equations (5.18) and (5.20) was *based on equilibrium* conditions. As the drug concentration in plasma water is reduced by renal and other mechanisms of reduction, the equilibrium is upset. Bound drug molecules dissociate from the protein-binding sites and more drug is eliminated. If the excretory mechanisms are sufficiently slow then the equilibrium conditions of Equations (5.18) and (5.20) will prevail, and *these equations may be used, but only as an approximate guide in determining the fraction bound.*\*

The most important consequences of protein binding are, first, the limitation of access to receptors†; second, the effect of this phenomenon on elimination rate; third, binding to plasma proteins is nonselective, i.e., there may be competition between drugs for the same protein-binding site, resulting in a displacement of one by the other; fourth, drugs that bind strongly to plasma protein usually also bind to other tissues, thus increasing the capacity of the "total depot." Aspects of protein binding that are related to the therapeutic usefulness

---

\* For example, Equation (5.20) says that as $(D) \to 0$, the fraction $r$ increases. Such an increase may happen transiently, but it should be obvious that a significant change in $(D)$ has upset the equilibrium and dissociation must now take place.

† Protein binding is often the reason for the low *potency* of a drug. For example, digitoxin is less potent than other cardiac glycosides because of its high binding to plasma proteins. All cardiac glycosides probably have the same *intrinsic activity* and *affinity*. The latter terms are related to the drug–receptor interaction in contrast to *potency* (see Chap. 3).

of drugs will be illustrated for a class of antibiotics discussed below. Finally, it should be mentioned that most analytic methods for determining drug concentration in blood do not distinguish between free and unbound drug, thus confounding the determination of many clinically useful measures such as hepatic clearance.[44,64]

## Antibiotic Therapy

Although protein binding occurs with many drugs, this phenomenon is particularly prevalent among some classes of antibiotics. These agents, therefore, illustrate the principles discussed previously. Another reason for selecting antibiotics as an example is that the expression of a dose–response relation for these agents is somewhat different, as we will see.

We have said previously the depot action resulting from protein binding prevents large fluctuations of the free drug in the body fluids; protein binding has been described, therefore, as a dynamic process.[40] Other actions of protein binding on antibiotics are, however, poorly understood,[47] for it is known that only the free antibiotic can exert its antibacterial action. Also antibiotics differ greatly in the degree of protein binding, both from one class to another and even within a class. This difference is illustrated in Table 5.4 for the cephalosporin group, an important group because of their widespread use.

**Table 5.4**
Protein binding of cephalosporins[a]

| Agent | % |
|-------|-----|
| Cephalothin[b] | 60 |
| Cephaloridine | 20 |
| Cephaloglycin | 10 |
| Cephalexin | 15 |
| Cefazolin | 86 |
| Cephapirin | 70 |
| Cefamandole | 74 |
| Cefoxitin | 70 |
| Cephradine | 15 |
| Cephacetrile | 40 |

[a] From Neu[40] with permission of the Southern Med. J.
[b] Reported as 70% by Neu.

Two popular agents within this group are cephalothin and cefazolin. Both of these have essentially the same antimicrobial spectrum,[39] but the pharmacokinetics of the two agents are different. Cefazolin is 86% protein bound whereas cephalothin is 60% to 70% bound. (Differences in the percent binding, reported by different workers when studying the same drug, are probably attributable to other variables such as the pH, the protein concentration, and the presence

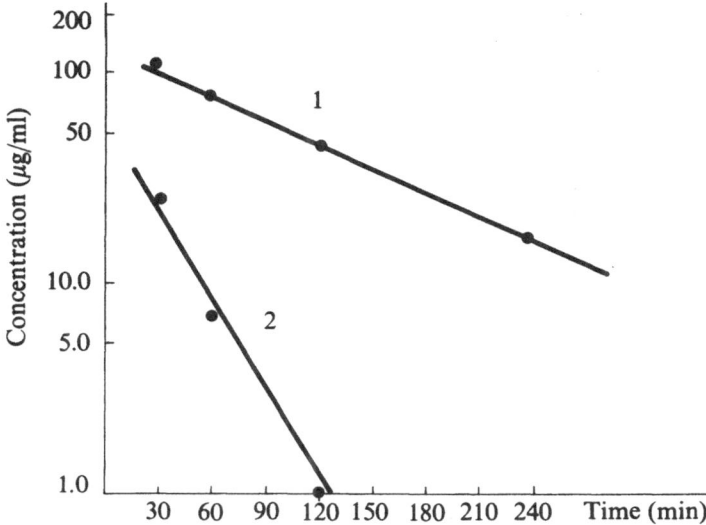

**Figure 5.7** Average serum concentration (micrograms per milliliter) as a function of time (minutes) after a single intravenous injection of 1 g for cefazolin (curve 1) and cephalothin (curve 2). (Data provided by Smith, Kline & French Laboratories.)

of other agents during the determination.) The high protein binding of these and other members of this class will, of course, affect the pharmacokinetics of these agents and, accordingly, the dosage schedule. Lipid solubility is also an important factor with drugs of this class; for example, cephalexin (an oral cephalosporin), which is only 15% protein bound, is not detectable in the cerebrospinal fluid.

The greater degree of protein binding of cefazolin (86%) over that of cephalothin (60%) results in the expected order relation between their half-lives of elimination from serum: 83 min for cefazolin and 23 min for cephalothin (Fig. 5.7). Hence, cefazolin is administered (for moderately severe infections) in a dose of 1 g every 8 hr. Cephalothin, on the other hand, is given in this same dose every 4 hr. There are obvious advantages with less frequent administration, namely, reduction in cost and decreased incidence of side effects, such as phlebitis and generalized tissue reactions that may accompany parenteral administration.

It is reasonable to ask whether appreciable protein binding reduces the overall effectiveness of the antibiotic since the bound drug is inactive. A reasonable answer is that the ultimate determinant of effectiveness is the amount of free drug present, and whether this amount is sufficient to destroy the infecting microorganism. The amount of drug necessary for destruction will depend upon the organism. An accurate method used involves inoculation of the micro-organism being tested into a liquid culture medium containing serial dilutions of the drug. One then determines the minimum concentration of the drug that

**Table 5.5**

Minimum inhibitory concentrations[a] of cefazolin and cephalothin[b]

|  | Cefazolin | Cephalothin |
|---|---|---|
| S. aureus (penicillin-sensitive) | 0.25 | 0.25 |
| S. aureus (penicillin-resistant) | 0.5 | 0.5 |
| E. coli | 1.6 | 6.3 |
| Klebsiella spp. | 1.0 | 2.0 |
| P. mirabilis | 6.3 | 4.0 |
| P. morganii | Res. | Res. |
| P. rettgeri | 32 | Res. |
| P. vulgaris | 64 | Res. |
| H. influenzae | 12.5 | 12.5 |
| B. fragilis | Res. | Res. |
| Enterobacter aerogenes | 2.0 | 5.0 |

[a] Micrograms per milliliter.
[b] Data supplied by Smith, Kline & French Laboratories.

inhibits the growth of the bacteria. This concentration is called the *minimum inhibitory concentration* (MIC) and is usually expressed in micrograms per milliliter. Table 5.5 gives the MICs of cefazolin and cephalothin for a number of microorganisms. A "MIC" table is, therefore, an expression of a dose-response relationship for antibiotic drugs. Such a table is used along with the average serum concentration in order to determine the dosage schedule. Cephalothin is eliminated largely in unchanged form by renal tubular secretion and, hence, its excretion rate is independent of its protein binding. However, cefazolin is eliminated from the body mainly by renal glomerular filtration, thus accounting for its slower rate of elimination.

## Receptor Status and Disease States

Improved techniques of analysis in recent years, especially progress in the use of radiolabeled materials, have produced a number of investigations aimed at correlating abnormal physiological states with changes in receptors. It would seem quite reasonable to assume that certain clinical conditions might be related to alterations in the concentration of receptors which interact with endogenous agents, or to changes in affinity of the agents for their specific receptors. For example, essential hypertension *might* be due to alterations in adrenoreceptors; obesity and ketotic diabetes (with the accompanying insulin resistance) *might* be due to changes in the insulin receptor; diseases affecting skeletal muscle action *might* be due to changes in neuromuscular postsynaptic or central receptors; and narcotic dependence and tolerance *might possibly* result from changes in the number or structure of opiate receptors.

The number of investigations aimed at answering such questions is increasing continually. Definitive answers to the above hypotheses do not exist at present, but a great deal of information is rapidly accumulating. For some disease states the information about altered receptors fits together better than it does in others.

The phenomenon of tolerance to the effects of morphine and morphine surrogates has been the focus of attention in a large number of studies conducted over the past several decades. It was once thought that tolerance might result from altered absorption, distribution, metabolism, or excretion. The main body of evidence, however, indicates that these mechanisms do not appear essential to the mechanisms of tolerance (see, for examples, the articles by Cochin[8,9]). Hence, attention in recent years has been directed at the in vivo receptor occupation by opiates and comparing the occupation to pharmacological effects.[23] To take a specific example of work in this field, we can point to the work of Bläsig and co-workers.[6] They studied the relative affinities of a set of morphine antagonists and partial agonists in order to determine their relative affinities for the opiate receptor. These investigators found that the order relation of receptor affinities of the several agents studied correlated well with their potencies in precipitating withdrawal in tolerant/dependent animals. This work is just one example. Work in this field is proceeding at such a rapid pace that probably by the time this is read many other investigations of the relationship of tolerance and dependence to receptor characteristics will have been conducted.

To turn to another area, hypertension, a receptor-linked mechanism has not been found, although several ingenious animal models have been employed for such studies. In one such study[65] desoxycorticosterone hypertensive rats were compared with normotensive rats in order to see whether there was a difference between the adrenergic receptors of each. Competitive inhibition to norepinephrine by phentolamine was measured in terms of the $pA_2$. No significant difference in the $pA_2$ values could be found. In a related study[26] another group looked at the number of $\alpha$-adrenergic receptors in aortic tissue from normotensive and genetically hypertensive rats. No difference in the estimated number of receptors could be detected.

Rather interesting work in humans has resulted in some new ideas in regard to the mechanism of myasthenia gravis, a disease affecting the neuromuscular junction. Recent evidence suggests that this condition is related to a reduction in the number of functional acetylcholine receptors in the postsynaptic membrane and not to diminished release of acetylcholine, as previously thought.[12]

Equally interesting are the studies of dopaminergic receptor states in patients with Parkinson's disease. Lee and co-workers[31] studied the postmortem brains of Parkinson patients with the use of [³H]haloperidol and [³H]-apomorphine as labels. They found increased haloperidol binding in the putamen of the untreated patient sample, presumably reflecting an increased number (or increased affinity constant) of postsynaptic dopamine receptors. This finding suggests that a phenomenon such as denervation supersensitivity occurs in Parkinson's disease, perhaps a compensatory factor in this disease.

Of all the disease states in which receptor alteration has been linked or suspected, diabetes has produced the most definitive findings. There is now an abundance of information regarding the status of the insulin receptor both in the normal and in the diabetic patient.[3] We now strongly suspect that there are alterations in the insulin receptor in this condition, particularly among obese insulin-resistant patients. Studies with $^{125}$I-labeled insulin have shown that many obese patients have impaired insulin-receptor binding and that long-term low-calorie dieting can improve the insulin binding.[2] In obese adult diabetes, elevated levels of insulin are common, a finding which is associated with insulin resistance and a decrease in receptor concentration.[4] Among thin diabetics, basal hyperinsulinemia is not very common, but, when present, is associated with a decrease in the concentration of insulin receptors.[42] (For further information see the review by Olefsky.[41])

Most likely, future studies of the kind described will help unravel the complexities of these and other disease states.

# References

1. Akera, T.: Science, *198*:569, 1977.
2. Archer, J. A., Gorden, P., and Roth, J.: J. Clin. Invest., *55*:166, 1975.
3. Bar, R. S., and Roth, J.: Arch. Intern. Med., **137**:474, 1977.
4. Bar, R. S., Gorden, P., and Roth, J: J. Clin. Invest., *58*:1123, 1976.
5. Barsoum, G. S., and Gaddum, J. H.: J. Physiol. (London), *85*:1, 1935.
6. Bläsig, J., Höllt, V., Herz, A., and Paschelke, G.: Psychopharmacologia, *46*:41, 1976.
7. Cantoni, G. L., and Eastman, G.: J. Pharmacol. Exp. Therap., *87*:392, 1946.
8. Cochin, J.: Fed. Proc., *29*:19, 1970.
9. Cochin, J. In *Drug Addiction, Experimental Pharmacology.* (Singh, J. M., Miller, L. and Lal, H. eds.) New York, Futura Publishing Co., 1972, p. 365.
10. Cowan, A., Tallarida, R. J., Maslow, J., and Adler, M. W.: Proc. 7th Int. Cong. Pharmacology, Paris, 1978, Abstracts, p. 168.
11. Cox, B. M.: Br. J. Pharmacol., *62*:387P, 1978.
12. Cull-Candy, S. G., Miledi, R., and Trautmann, A.: Nature, *271*:74, 1978.
13. Del Castillo, J., and Katz, B.: Proc. R. Soc. London, Ser., B *146*:369, 1957.
14. Dum, J., Meyer, G., Höllt, V., Herz, A., and Catlin, D. H.: Eur. J. Pharmacol., *46*:165, 1977.
15. Furchgott, R. F.: Fed. Proc., *37*:115, 1978.
16. Gero, A.: Arch. Int. Pharmacodyn., *206*:41, 1973.
17. Gero, A.: J. Mol. Medicine, *1*:161, 1976.
18. Giachetti, A., and Shore, P. A.: Life Sci., *23*:89, 1978.
19. Goldstein, A., Lowney, K. I., and Pal, B. K.: Proc. Natl. Acad. Sci. U.S.A., *68*:1742, 1971.
20. Guldberg, C. M., and Waage, P.: In *Physical Chemistry* (W. J. Moore, ed.), 4th ed. Englewood Cliffs, N.J., Prentice-Hall, 1972, p. 282.

21. Hayashi, G., and Takemori, A. E.: Eur. J. Pharmacol., *16*:63. 1971.
22. Hogben, C. A., Tocco, D. J., Brodie, B. B., and Schanker, L. S.: J. Pharmacol. Exp. Therap., *125*:275, 1959.
23. Höllt, V., and Herz, A.: Fed. Proc., *37*:158, 1978.
24. Höllt, V., Dum, J., Bläsig, J., Schubert, P., and Herz, A.: Life Sci., *16*:1823, 1975.
25. Hulme, E. C., Birdsall, N. J. M., Burgen, A. S. V., and Mehta, P.: Mol. Pharmacol., *14*:737, 1978.
26. Janis, R. A., and Triggle, D. J.: J. Pharmacol. Exp. Therap., *24*:602, 1972.
27. Katz, B., and Thesleff, S.: J. Physiol. (London), *138*:63, 1957.
28. Kebabian, J. W., and Calne, D. B.: Nature *277*:93, 1979.
29. Koshland, D. E.: Fed. Proc., *23*:719, 1964.
30. La Du, B. N., Mandel, H. G., and Way, E. L.: *Fundamentals of Drug Metabolism and Disposition.* Baltimore, Williams and Wilkins, 1971.
31. Lee, T., Seeman, P., Rajput, A., Farley, I. J., and Hornykiewicz, O.: Nature, *273*:59, 1978.
32. Loh, H. L., Law, P. Y., Ostwald, T., Cho, T. M., and Way, E. L.: Fed. Proc., *37*:147, 1978.
33. Lullman, H., and Ziegler, A.: Naunyn-Schmiedebergs Arch. Pharmacol., *280*:1, 1973.
34. Martin, W. R., Eades, C. G., Thompson, J. A., Huppler, R. E., and Gilbert, P. E.: J. Pharmacol. Exp. Therap., *197*:517, 1976.
35. McGilliard, K. L., Tulunay, F. C., and Takemori, A. E.: In *Opiates and Endogenous Opioid Peptides* (H. W. Kosterlitz, ed.) Amsterdam, North Holland Publishing Co., 1976, p. 281.
36. McGilliard, K., and Takemori, A. E.: J. Pharmacol. Exp. Ther., *207*:884, 1978.
37. MacNab, M. W. Ph.D. Thesis, Temple University Medical School, Philadelphia, Pa., 1974.
38. Möhler, H., and Okada, T.: Science, *198*:849, 1977.
39. Mollering, R. C., and Swartz, M. N.: Drug Therapy, *4*:85, 1976.
40. Neu, H. C.: Southern Med. J., *70* (Supp. 1):14, 1977.
41. Olefsky, J. M.: Diabetes, *25*:1154, 1976.
42. Olefsky, J. M., and Reaven, G. M.: J. Clin. Invest., *54*:1323, 1975.
43. Pert, C. B., and Snyder, S. H.: Science, *179*:1011, 1973.
44. Rane, A., Wilkinson, G. R., and Shand, D. G.: J. Pharmacol. Exp. Therap., *200*:420, 1977.
45. Rang, H. P., and Ritter, J. M.: Mol. Pharmacol., *6*:357, 1970.
46. Riggs, D. S.: *The Mathematical Approach to Physiological Problems.* Baltimore, Williams and Wilkins, 1963.
47. Robinson, G. N., and Sutherland, R.: Br. J. Pharmacol., *25*:638, 1965.
48. Schanker, L. S.: Ann. Rev. Pharmacol., *1*:29, 1961.
49. Shen, J. W., and Way, E. L.: Life Sci., *16*:77, 1975.
50. Simon, E. J., and Hiller, J. M.: Ann. Rev. Pharmacol. Toxicol., *18*:371, 1978.
51. Simon, E. J., and Hiller, J. M.: Fed. Proc., *37*:141, 1978.
52. Smits, S. E., and Takemori, A. E.: Br. J. Pharmacol., *39*:627, 1970.
53. Stahl, K. D., Van Bever, W., Janssen, P., and Simon, E. J.: Eur. J. Pharmacol., *46*:199, 1977.
54. Szekely, J. I., Dunai-Kovacs, Z., Miglecz, E., Ronai, A. Z., and Bajusz, S.: J. Pharmacol. Exp. Ther., *207*:878, 1978.
55. Takemori, A. E.: In *Narcotic Antagonists.* M. C. Braude, L. S. Harris, E. L. May, J. P. Smith, and J. E. Villarreal, eds. Advances in Biochemical Psychopharmacology, *8*, New York, Raven Press, 1974, p. 335.
56. Tallarida, R. J., Cowan, A., and Adler, M. W.: Life Sciences, *25*:637, 1979.
57. Tallarida, R. J., Harakal, C., Rusy, B. F., and Sevy, R. W.: Currents in Modern Biol., *2*:249, 1968.
58. Tallarida, R. J., Harakal, C., Maslow, J., Geller, E. B., and Adler, M. W.: J. Pharmacol. Exp. Ther., *206*:38, 1978.
59. Terenius, L.: Acta Pharmacol. Toxicol., *32*:317, 1973.
60. Tsai, B. S., and Lefkowitz, R. J.: J. Pharmacol. Exp. Therap., *204*:606, 1978.
61. Tulunay, F. C.: In *Characteristics and Function of Opioids* (G. M. Van Ree, and L. Terenius, eds.) Amsterdam, Elsevier-North Holland, 1978, p. 495.

62. Wagner, J. G.: *Biopharmaceutics* and *Relevant Pharmacokinetics*. Hamilton, Ill., 1971. Drug Intelligence Publications, 1971.
63. Waud, D. R.: Pharmacol. Rev., *20*:49, 1968.
64. Wilkinson, G. R., and Schenker, S.: Biochem. Pharmacol., *25*:2675, 1976.
65. Wohl, A. J., Hausler, L. M., and Roth, F. E.: J. Pharmacol. Exp. Therap., *162*:109, 1968.
66. Yaksh, T. L., and Rudy, T. A.: J. Pharmacol. Exp. Therap., *202*:411, 1977.

# Isolated Preparations: Dose–Response Data

## Chapter 6

Much of our practical knowledge of pharmacology and many of the theories of drug action have been attained from experiments conducted on isolated preparations. When we work with isolated preparations we can observe the direct actions of drugs on the organ of interest. These observations are reasonably unencumbered by the many compensatory mechanisms of the organism that often mask the drugs' direct actions. Yet, working at this level, we remain within the realm of investigation that permits us to connect observations on the whole animal with the more intimate action of drugs on individual molecules. In this chapter we discuss several of these isolated preparations and present dose–response data for selected agents which act on them.

### Rabbit Thoracic Aorta

There are a variety of in vitro preparations for studying the effects of drugs on vascular smooth muscle. The reader is referred to several extensive reviews that summarize much of the experimental work on the various preparations.[9,26,58,59]

One of the most frequently used preparations is the isolated thoracic aorta of the rabbit. Drug effects on this preparation are both direct and indirect. Direct action results from interaction of the drug with a specific receptor; indirect action results from effects on nonreceptor components of the cell, resulting in the release of or accumulation of a substance that has direct action. Having discussed in general the concept of specific receptors for specific drugs, we now present information on some drugs most often used in pharmacological studies which employ this preparation.

Epinephrine is known to produce both contraction and relaxation of vascular smooth muscle, and both effects are seen in the rabbit aorta. The most common effect is contraction,[39] an effect mediated through the interaction of epinephrine with the α-adrenergic receptor.[1] The relaxation produced by epinephrine is mediated through the β-adrenergic receptor.[1] Norepinephrine is similar in its effect on this preparation, acting on both α- and β-receptors. The potency of norepinephrine for the inhibitory β-receptors, however, is less than that of epinephrine for these receptors; hence, the relaxation produced by norepinephrine is less prominent than that of epinephrine. Norepinephrine, however, produces constriction of vascular smooth muscle at lower doses than epinephrine,[27] indicating that the potency of norepinephrine for the α-receptor is higher than that of epinephrine. The actions of both these amines are illustrated in Figures 6.1 and 6.2. The dose–response curve for angiotensin II on this preparation is shown in Figure 6.3.

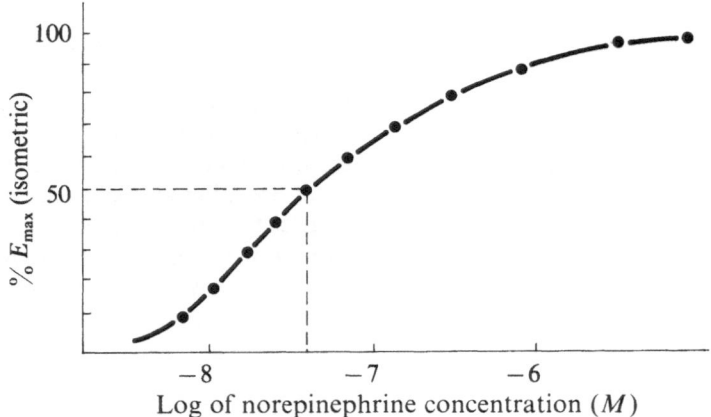

**Figure 6.1** Dose–response relation for norepinephrine on rabbit aortic strips.[60] (Reprinted with permission of IEEE Trans. Biomed. Engineering.)

Histamine and serotonin constrict the rabbit thoracic aorta (Figs. 6.4, 6.5). Each of these agents acts through its own specific receptor, a fact which is known from experiments conducted with specific antagonists of each as discussed in Chapter 3. The differentiation of the receptors for histamine and serotonin from the α-adrenergic receptors may be illustrated by treating the preparation with a specific α-antagonist such as dibenamine.[28]

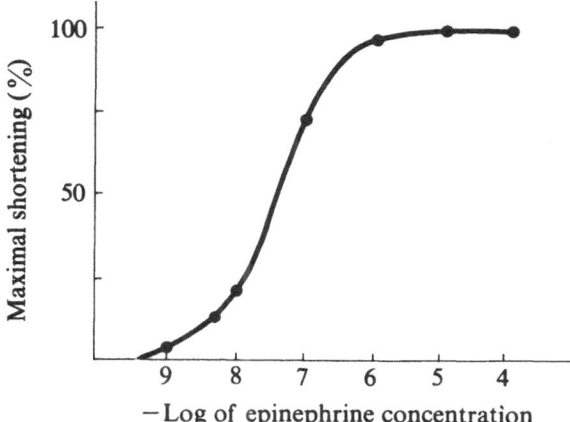

**Figure 6.2** Dose–response relation for epinephrine on rabbit aortic strips.[28] (Reprinted with permission of J. Pharmacol. Exp. Therap.)

The rabbit thoracic aorta serves as a diverse pharmacological preparation useful in classifying both agonist and antagonist effects in vascular smooth muscle. Some details of the methods of preparation and results of experimentation with various drugs are given below.

### Method of Preparation

The most consistent results are seen in aortic strips taken from mature albino rabbits weighing 2.5–3.5 kg. The animal is killed either by a blow on the head, cervical dislocation, or a rapid intravenous injection of sodium pentobarbital

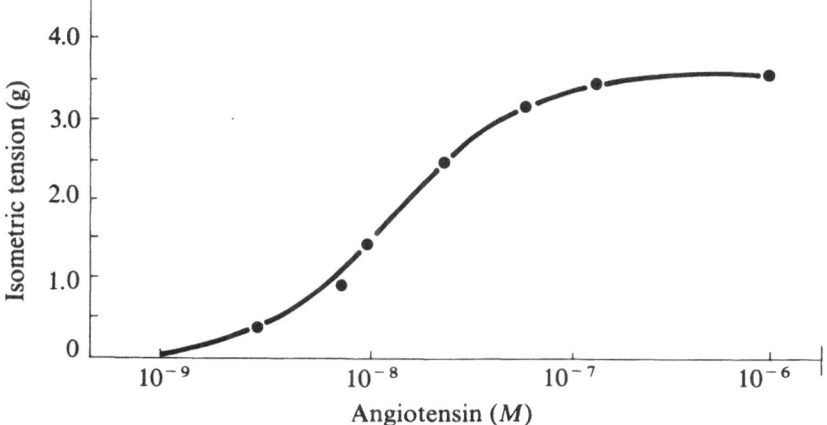

**Figure 6.3** Dose–response relation for angiotensin II on rabbit aortic strips.[33] (Reprinted with permission of Arch. Int. Pharmacodyn.)

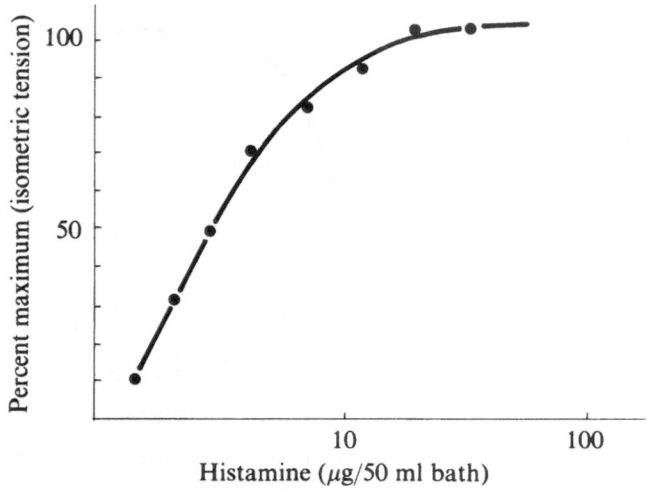

**Figure 6.4** Dose–response relation for histamine on rabbit aortic strips.[46]

(60 mg/kg). The chest cavity is opened and the descending thoracic aorta is quickly removed and placed in a solution of Krebs-bicarbonate plus glucose (see Appendix B, Table B.2, for composition). Fat and connective tissue should be removed while keeping the preparation moistened with the solution. Rings of approximately 2.5-mm width are cut, producing a rectangular strip when opened. The length of a typical strip is 12 mm, and its thickness is 0.4 mm. The entire procedure of strip preparation may be carried out at room temperature.

The prepared strip is placed in a muscle chamber containing the solution mentioned previously. Several methods of mounting exist, depending on whether isotonic or isometric recording is to be employed.[29] Improvements in

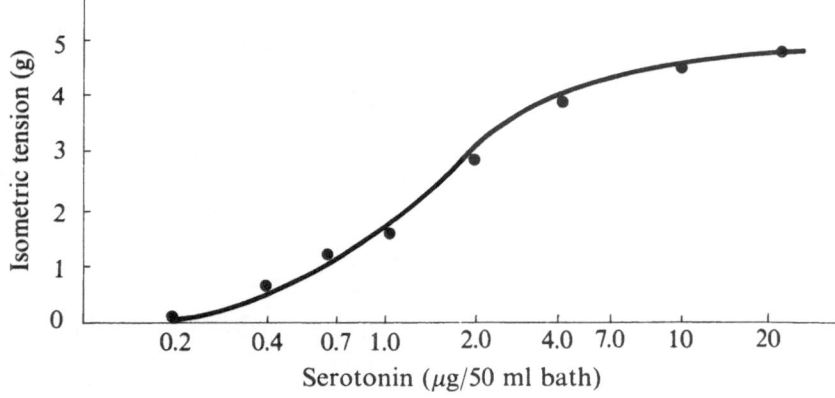

**Figure 6.5** Dose–response relation for serotonin on rabbit aortic strips. (Data supplied by Dr. C. Harakal, Temple University Medical School.)

instrumentation in recent years have resulted in considerable variability in mounting and in methods of recording. A satisfactory method used by the authors employs the use of thin gold chains with small plastic clamps for isometric recording. The two ends of the muscle strip are attached to the plastic clamps. The shorter bottom chain contains a loop which slips over a stationary L-shaped glass rod. The longer chain connects the upper end of the muscle strip to an isometric force transducer; an S-hook may be used to connect the chain to the force transducer. The transducer is electrically connected to an appropriate recording device, such as strip chart recorder or oscilloscope. It is important that, during the mounting, the muscle not be stretched excessively since mechanical trauma can kill the muscle.

When experimenting with epinephrine and norepinephrine, propranolol ($2 \times 10^{-6}$ $M$) and cocaine ($2 \times 10^{-5}$ $M$) are added to the bathing solution. Propranolol blocks $\beta$-receptors; cocaine prevents neuronal reuptake into storage sites.

The bath is maintained at 37°C and is aerated with a mixture of 95% $O_2$ and 5% $CO_2$. The pH of the solution is 7.4.

Prior to dosing, the muscle should be stretched by the application of a preload mass of 10 g while in the bathing solution at constant temperature. In the isometric mount described above this preloading procedure is accomplished by increasing the tension until the force transducer reads 10 g. As the muscle lengthens under this load, the tension will fall, requiring continual restoration of the preload to 10 g. Equilibration under the preload should take place for at least 2 hr before drugs are administered. This tension-time period permits stabilization of the muscle and results in maximal drug sensitivity. The bath should be changed after 1 hr and just prior to dosing.

## Guinea Pig Ileum

The guinea pig ileum is the most frequently used of the in vitro preparations for evaluating drug action on intestinal smooth muscle. Unlike isolated intestine of other species (e.g., the rabbit) that exhibit spontaneous contracture, the guinea pig ileum shows little spontaneous activity. This preparation is suitable, therefore, for viewing drug-induced changes in muscle tension.

Because of the anatomic location of parasympathetic ganglia, the excised ileum contains the ganglia, the postganglionic neuron, the cholinergic (muscarinic) receptor, and certain other drug receptors. Hence, agents that stimulate ganglia through interaction with "nicotine I" receptors would be expected to contract this preparation by effecting release of acetylcholine.[63] Certainly, muscarinic agents will contract the guinea pig ileum by direct combination with the postganglionic cholinergic receptor, as will other agents having specific receptors in the muscle (Figs. 6.6, 6.7).

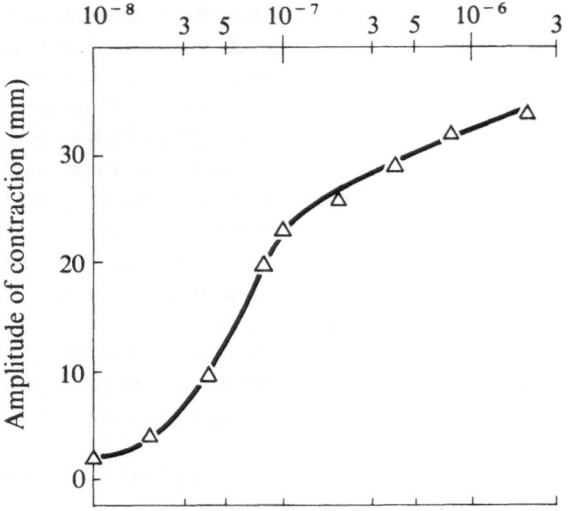

**Figure 6.6** Dose–response relation for acetylcholine on guinea pig ileum.[7] (Reprinted with permission of Br. J. Pharmacol.)

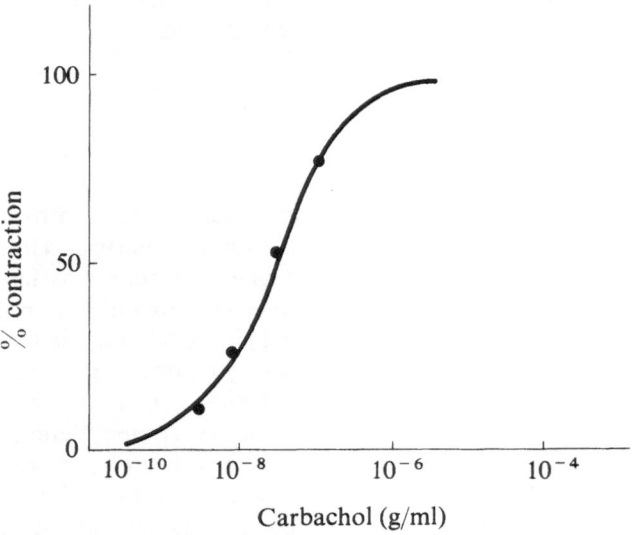

**Figure 6.7** Dose–response relation for carbachol on guinea pig ileum.[16] (Reprinted with permission of Br. J. Pharmacol.)

Small doses of acetylcholine are known to have nicotinic action.[23,24] Such action stimulates the ganglia of the ileum (Auerbach's plexus) promoting release of acetylcholine from the postganglionic neuron. Thus, there are two components to acetylcholine's action in contracting this preparation. Experiments with ganglionic blockers, such as hexamethonium, and with the muscarinic blockers, atropine and hyoscine, permit a comparison of the relative contributions of the two components of acetylcholine action. The results of such experiments indicate that the muscarinic action is the more important of the two components. The action of nicotine on this preparation is shown in the dose–response curve of Figure 6.8.

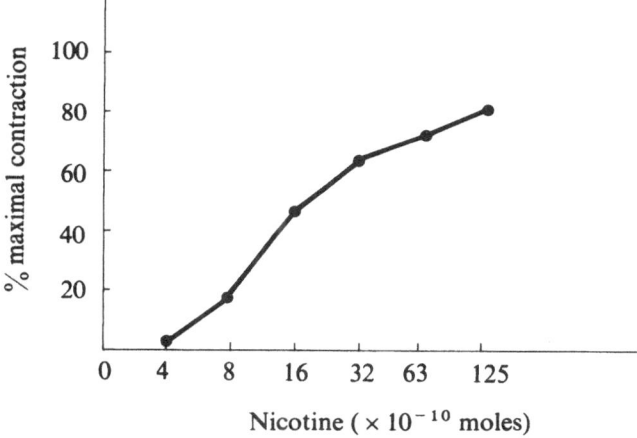

Figure 6.8  Dose–response relation for nicotine on guinea pig ileum.[57] (Reprinted with permission of J. Pharmacol. Exp. Therap.)

Carbamylcholine, a parasympathomimetic agent, is frequently used instead of acetylcholine in experiments on the ileum. It is less susceptible to the hydrolyzing cholinesterase enzymes,[37] an advantage over acetylcholine. In all other respects the action of carbamylcholine on the guinea pig ileum is similar to that of acetylcholine.

Histamine contracts the guinea pig ileum (Fig. 6.9). For a long time the existence of a specific histamine receptor in the ileum could not be firmly established. The reason for the uncertainty is due to the fact that pure histamine antagonists have anticholinergic action and anticholinergics have antihistamine action. This duality precluded the use of the usual experiment that employs specific blockers to answer the question of one or two receptors. As mentioned in the discussion of competitive antagonism in Chapter 3, and now applied to histamine, a pure competitive antagonist of histamine should shift the dose–response curve of histamine to the right and have no affect on the dose–response

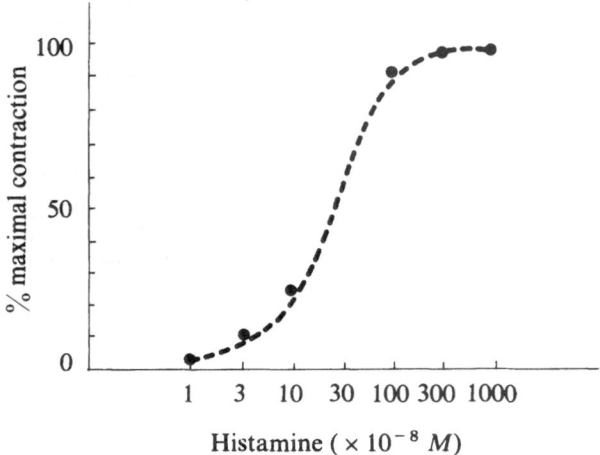

**Figure 6.9** Dose–response relation for histamine on guinea pig ileum.[57] (Reprinted with permission of J. Pharmacol. Exp. Therap.)

curve of acetylcholine, *if each agonist has its own specific receptor.* Since, however, the antihistamine is also anticholinergic, such an experiment is inconclusive.

Gero and Gurland[31] examined this question by using a method of analysis previously used by Gero[30] for distinguishing whether one or two receptors exist. Gero's method utilized isobolar plots of the type discussed in Chapter 1. As applied to the case in question, Gero and Gurland used histamine and furtrethonium (a cholinergic drug) and plotted loci of identical effects. They concluded that the receptor for histamine in the ileum is specific and distinct from the acetylcholine receptor. The effect of histamine is contraction. Van Den Brink and Lien[61] used this preparation in a very extensive study of the affinity and intrinsic activity of a number of histaminergic agents.

Prostaglandins $E_1$ and $E_2$ affect intestinal activity both in vitro and in vivo[6] (Fig. 6.10). Serosal application of prostaglandin to isolated guinea pig ileum stimulates longitudinal muscle, but the peristaltic contractions of the circular muscle are reduced. Intraluminal application of prostaglandin has no discernable effect. Serotonin produces contraction in this preparation (Fig. 6.11).

The effects of inhibitory drugs cannot be obviously demonstrated in an intestine which lacks active tension. For example, when catecholamines are administered to the isolated guinea pig ileum which is stretched passively, there is no reduction in tension. Drug-induced relaxation must be preceded by active tension. This can be achieved either by excitatory drugs or by the technique of co-axial electrical stimulation.[50] The method consists of passing current pulses from one electrode in the bath fluid, in which a piece of guinea pig ileum is suspended, to another within the lumen of the gut. Twitches of the longitudinal

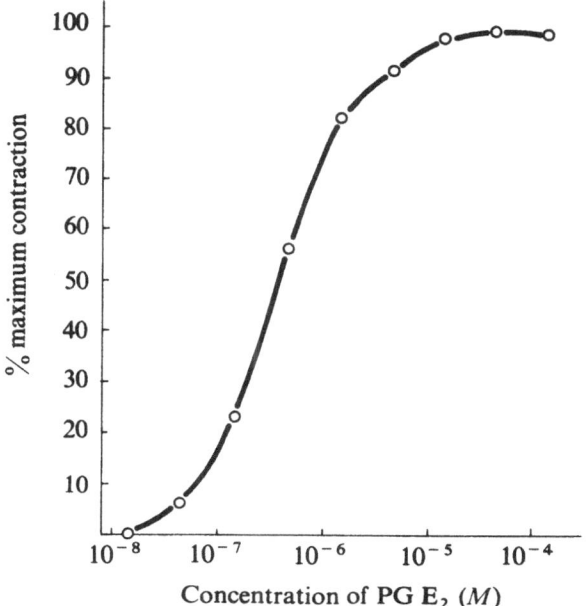

**Figure 6.10** Dose–response relation for prostaglandin $E_2$ on guinea pig ileum.[55] (Reprinted with permission of Arch. Int. Pharmacodyn.)

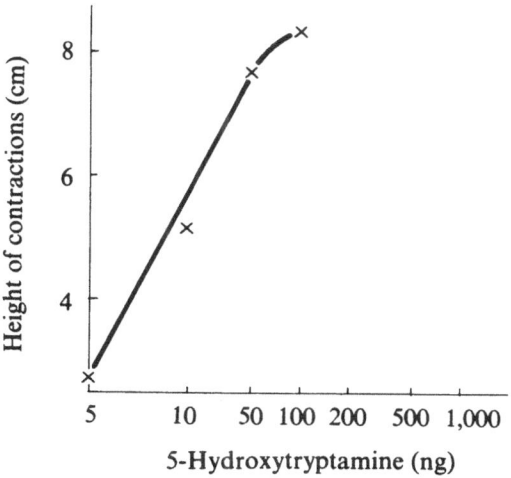

**Figure 6.11** Dose–response relation for 5-hydroxytryptamine (serotonin) on guinea pig ileum.[5] (Reprinted with permission of Br. J. Pharmacol.)

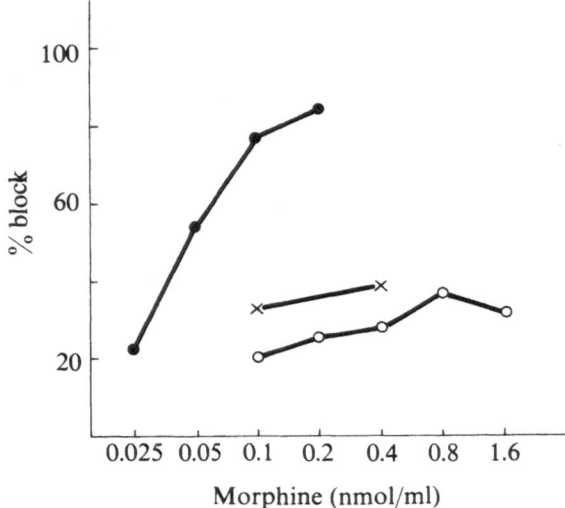

**Figure 6.12** Dose–response relation for morphine on the guinea pig ileum. The effect is the inhibition of acetylcholine release in the electrically stimulated ileum and is plotted on the ordinate as percent reduction in contraction height. The abscissa is the concentration of morphine in nanomoles per milliliter. ○, stimulus 500 μs, 20 V, giving maximal contractions; ●, stimulus 60 μs, 20 V, giving submaximal contractions; x, stimulus 60 μs, 60 V, giving maximal contractions.[21] (Reprinted with permission of Br. J. Pharmacol.)

muscle in response to single stimuli of 50 μs duration can be obtained; such twitches are augmented and prolonged by eserine, and insensitive to hexamethonium and nicotine, are reduced by procaine, and are abolished by small doses of atropine. Paton[50] concluded from the character of the strength–duration curve and from the pharmacological responses that the nerves supplying the muscles are stimulated.

In a study on the action of morphine, Paton[51] found that this narcotic depresses both the twitch caused by a single electrical stimulus and the tetanic response produced by repetitive stimulation. Dose–response curves for this action of morphine, obtained by Cox and Weinstock,[21] are shown in Figure 6.12. Other morphine-like drugs also reduce the size of the twitch, their relative potencies being related to their analgesic potencies. The analysis of the action of morphine is complicated by the fact that the ileum rapidly develops tolerance to morphine and morphine-like drugs. The inhibitory action of morphine is *not due to a depression of the response* of the longitudinal muscle to acetylcholine.

Schaumann[56] demonstrated that the contractions of the longitudinal muscle caused by co-axial stimulation are inhibited not only by morphine-like drugs but also by norepinephrine and epinephrine; the effects of the catecholamines are antagonized by the adrenergic blockers phentolamine and tolazoline. The experimental method is now discussed.

## Method of Preparation

The method most commonly used is that of Magnus.[47] A guinea pig is killed by a blow on the head. The abdomen is opened and the cecum is lifted forward. The ileum is joined to the back of the cecum. A length of ileum (2 to 3 cm) is removed and placed in a dish containing Tyrode's solution (see Appendix B, Table B.2). Fecal contents are washed out by placing one end of the ileum over the tip of a pipette containing Tyrode's solution.

The terminal portion of the guinea pig ileum appears to be the most sensitive in response to drugs, though other regions may be used. Care should be taken to avoid damaging the ileal muscle. Forceps or other instruments are not recommended.

The tubular segment is suspended in the muscle chamber in either of two methods. In one method each end is tied with surgical thread, thus closing the lumen. In the other method, S-hooks are used to pierce each end of the tubular segment, thus keeping the lumen open to the bathing solution. The second method permits maximum surface area on which the drug can act and also seems to minimize spontaneous activity. Tyrode's solution is aerated with 95% $O_2$ and 5% $CO_2$.

Experiments are performed at either room temperature (25°C) or at 37°C. The most frequently used preload tension is 1 g. The equilibration period is 30 min. Several changes of the bath, approximately every 5 min, should precede the initial dosing. Both isotonic and isometric procedures have been used.

## Isolated Taenia Ceca

The taenia from the guinea pig cecum has proved to be a useful preparation in electrophysiological experimentation.[18] It has been employed in a variety of pharmacological experiments as well. Bülbring[13,15] described the effects of acetylcholine, histamine, and epinephrine on the membrane potential and recorded the tension produced by each in several studies. A classification of the receptors mediating responses in this muscle, however, is due to Akubue,[4] who conducted studies with several agonists and antagonists. Akubue found that contractions produced by nicotine were almost abolished by 0.005 g/ml of hyoscine (Fig. 6.13a) while those produced by acetylcholine and 5-HT were only reduced by this same dose of hyoscine (Fig. 6.13b,c). Responses to histamine were not affected by hyoscine (Fig. 6.13d). He concluded that nicotine or acetylcholine either directly or indirectly activated muscarinic receptors and that part of the response to 5-HT was located at this site. Akubue also demonstrated that the responses of smooth muscle to acetylcholine, nicotine, and 5-HT, but not those to histamine, were potentiated by the anticholinesterase agent mipafox (Fig. 6.14). He concluded that these findings were further evidence that the action of nicotine and 5-HT involved a cholinergic mechanism.

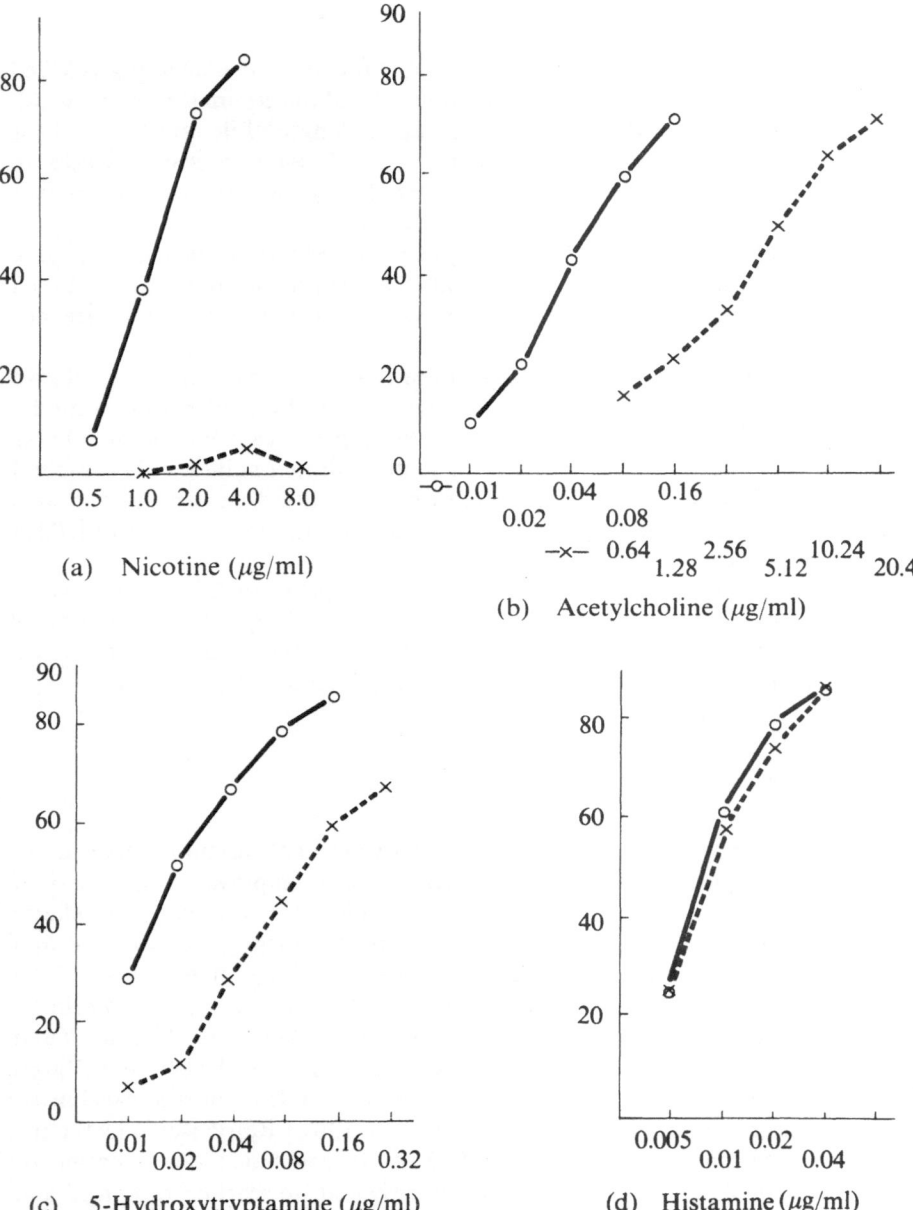

**Figure 6.13a–d**  Dose–response curves for several agonists (open circles) on the isolated taenia ceca of the guinea pig and the effect of the same fixed dose of hyoscine (0.005 μg/ml) on the dose–response curve of each agonist (crosses). The relations are expressed as percent of maximal contraction against the agonist concentration (μg/ml).[4] (Reprinted with permission of Br. J. Pharmacol.)

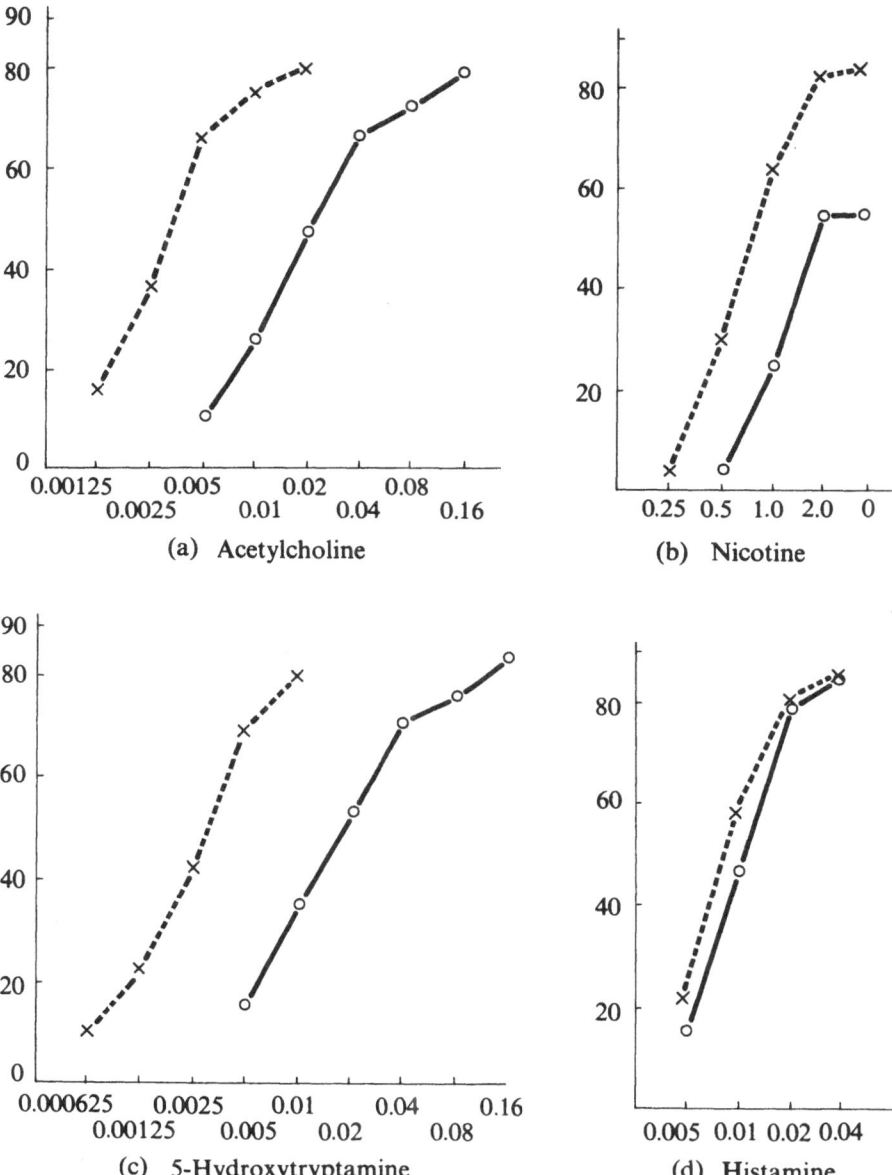

(a)  Acetylcholine

(b)  Nicotine

(c)  5-Hydroxytryptamine

(d)  Histamine

**Figure 6.14a–d**   The effect of treating the guinea pig taenia ceca with the anticholinesterase drug Mipafox (20 µg/ml) for 1 hr on the dose–response curve of each agonist. The open circles represent the responses to the agonists and the crosses represent the agonist dose–response curve after the treatment with Mipafox. Ordinate is calibrated as percent of the maximum contraction. The abscissa is the agonist concentration (µg/ml).[4] (Reprinted with permission of Br. J. Pharmacol.)

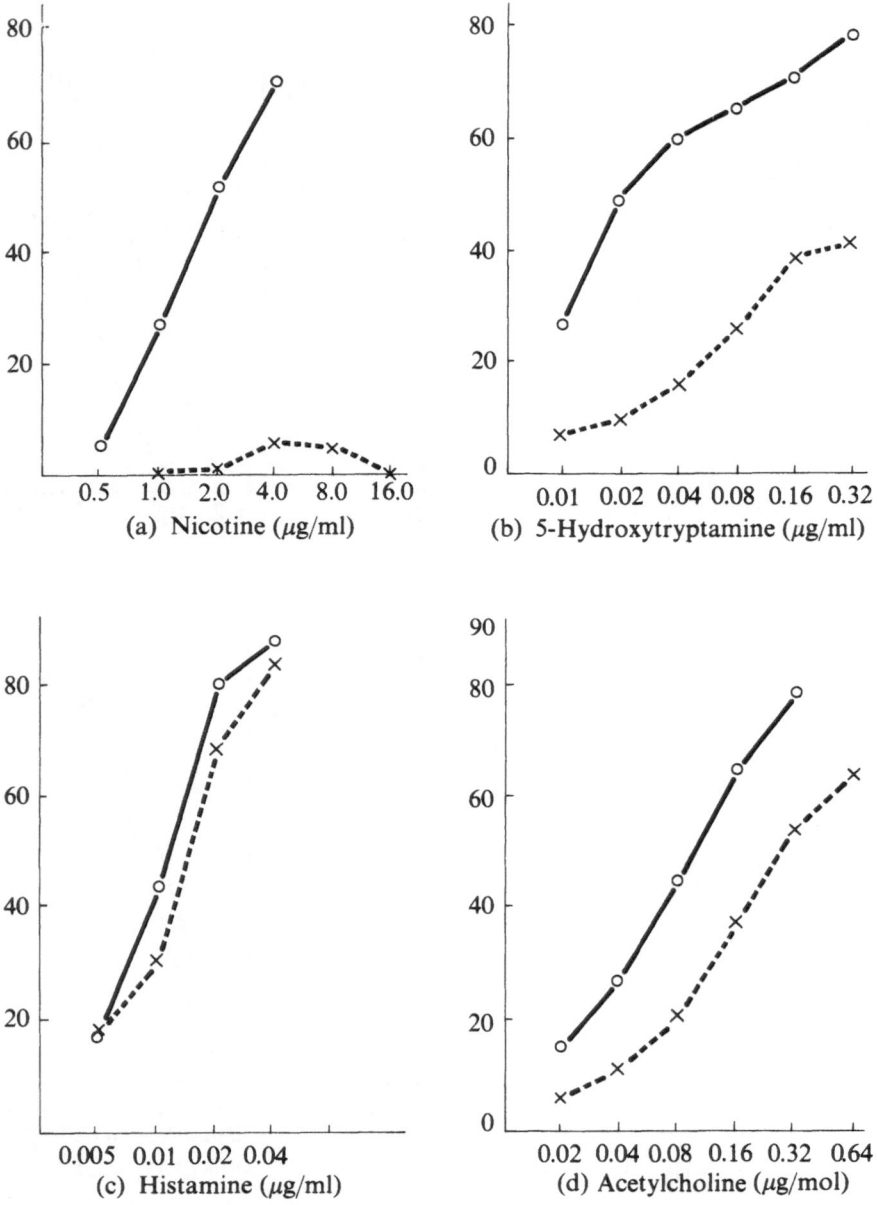

**Figure 6.15a–d** The effect of a fixed dose of procaine (10 μg/ml) on the responses of the guinea pig taenia ceca to several agonists. The open circles represent the responses to the agonists and the crosses represent the agonist dose–response curve in the presence of procaine. Ordinate is calibrated as percent of the maximum contraction. The abscissa is the agonist concentration (μg/ml).[4] (Reprinted with permission of Br. J. Pharmacol.)

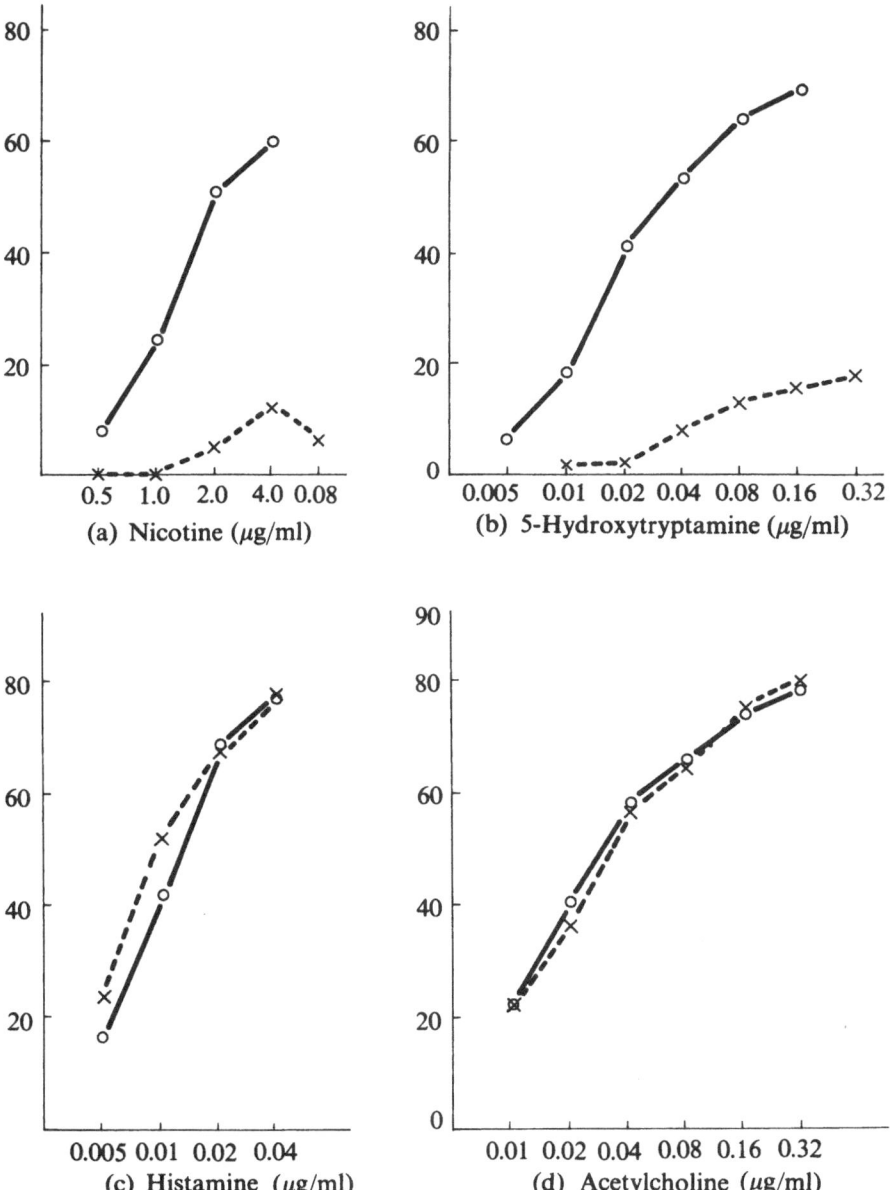

**Figure 6.16a–d** The effect of treating guinea pig taenia ceca with morphine (0.1 μg/ml) on the responses to several agonists. The open circles represent the responses to the agonists and the crosses represent the agonist dose–response curve in the presence of morphine. Ordinate is calibrated as percent of the maximum contraction. The abscissa is the agonist concentration (μg/ml).[4] (Reprinted with permission of Br. J. Pharmacol.)

Akubue also examined the effects of the local anesthetics, procaine and cocaine. These, he found, greatly abolished the responses to nicotine and reduced those to 5-HT, but they did not modify those to histamine. The antagonism by procaine is illustrated in Figure 6.15a–c. The effect of acetylcholine was only slightly reduced by procaine (Fig. 6.15d), but not by cocaine. Thus, it was reasoned that procaine might have an atropine-like action. Morphine antagonized the responses of the taenia to nicotine and 5-HT (Fig. 6.16a,b) but not those to histamine or acetylcholine (Fig. 6.16c,d).

It was concluded that acetylcholine or histamine activates receptors that are situated on smooth muscle cells, whereas nicotine stimulates ganglion cells (nicotinic I receptors). The actions of 5-HT were due in part to a direct effect on the smooth muscle and in part to stimulation of cholinergic ganglion cells.

### Method of Preparation (Modified from Bülbring[13])

The guinea pig is killed by a blow to the head. The abdomen is opened and the colon is exposed. The taenia are the longitudinal muscles that lie on a thin membrane that contains circular muscle fibers. A silk ligature is passed underneath the taenia and tied; the muscular coat is then cut beside this ligature, taking care not to penetrate the intestinal lumen. As the cut end of the taenia is lifted, the whole muscular coat, i.e., the membrane with the taenia on it, is separated by blunt dissection from the underlying submucosa and mucosa, the blood vessels remaining mostly undamaged. The preparation is then set up in an organ bath containing 10 ml of Krebs solution and kept at a constant temperature of 37°C. Both the bath solution and the solution in the reservoir are aerated with a mixture of 95% $O_2$ and 5% $CO_2$. The muscle is attached to a light lever for isotonic recording. The load on the tissue is set at 300 mg. An equilibration period of 30 min is required before dosing. Five washes should be made between experiments.

## Ductus Deferens Preparation of the Guinea Pig and Rat

The classic preparation consisting of the isolated guinea pig ductus deferens together with the sympathetic hypogastric nerve was described by Hukovic.[32] The ductus contracts in response to stimulation of the hypogastric nerve. The tissue will also contract in response to certain agents without stimulating the nerve. Birmingham[8] studied and compared the responses in both innervated and denervated rat vasa deferentia to agonist drugs. In most cases the guinea pig and rat preparations are quite similar. Both preparations will contract in response to epinephrine and norepinephrine, but their sensitivity appears to vary with the age of the animal. Younger animals are more sensitive.[42]

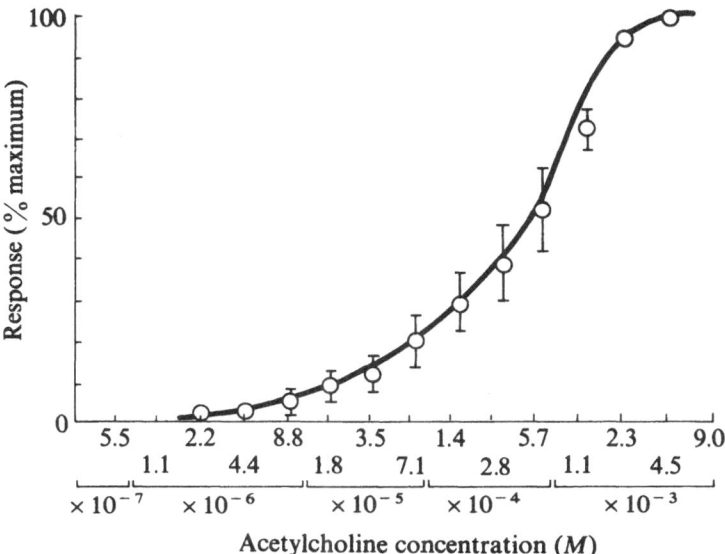

**Figure 6.17** Log concentration–response curve to acetylcholine for the mean responses of the vasa deferentia from four rats: The standard errors of the means are shown as vertical bars. Ordinate: contraction height as a percentage of the maximum response. Abscissa: final bath concentration $(M)$ of acetylcholine on a log scale.[8] (Reprinted with permission of Br. J. Pharmacol.)

The vas deferens will respond directly to acetylcholine, epinephrine, dopamine, and norepinephrine[8] as seen in Figures 6.17–6.20. Thus, like the rabbit aorta, this preparation can be used to test a variety of agents.

It is known that the sympathetic agonists are receptor specific because phentolamine will effectively block contractions induced by epinephrine and norepinephrine. Acetylcholine, which also causes contraction, is blocked by atropine. Thus, both $\alpha$-adrenergic and cholinergic muscarinic receptors are present. The effect of hypogastric nerve stimulation is not blocked by atropine, but it is blocked by substances that decrease release of its neurotransmitter. Since guanethidine and bretyllium will alter the response of the nerve to stimulation, and since this alteration can be effectively reversed by administration of epinephrine, the nerve terminal must be sympathetic. Some peripheral sympathetic ganglia are probably present in this preparation since hexamethonium, a ganglionic blocker, reduces the response of hypogastric stimulation.

## Method of Preparation[32]

The guinea pig or rat is killed by a blow to the head and bled out. The animal is then placed on its back. The abdomen is opened at the midline and the gut is

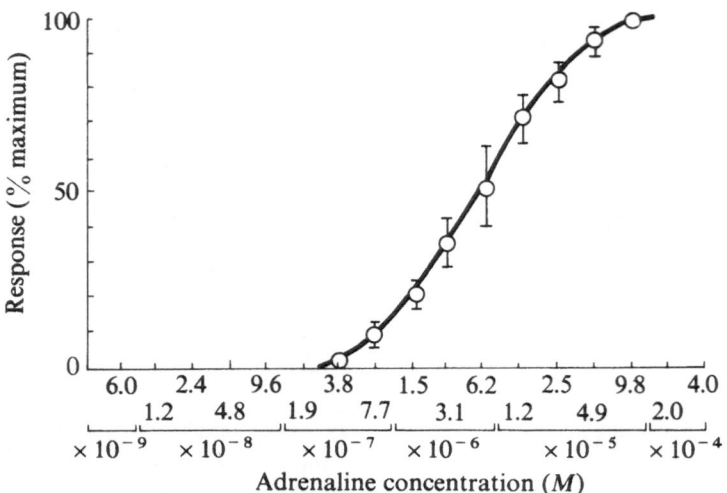

**Figure 6.18** Log concentration–response curve to (−)-adrenaline for the mean responses of the vasa deferentia from four rats; the standard errors of the means are shown as vertical bars. Ordinate: contraction height as a percentage of the maximum response. Abscissa: final bath concentration (M) of adrenaline on a log scale.[8] (Reprinted with permission of Br. J. Pharmacol.)

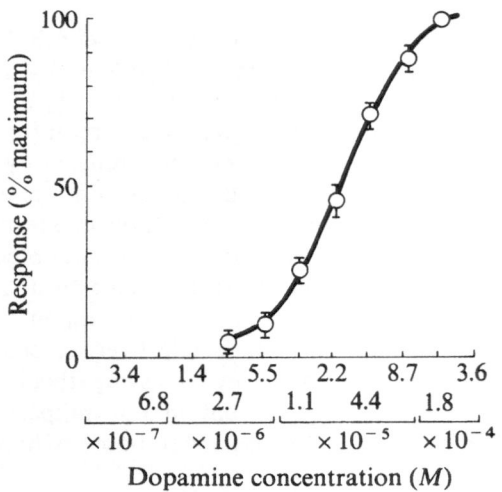

**Figure 6.19** Log concentration–response curve to dopamine for the mean responses of the vasa deferentia from four rats. The standard errors of the means are shown as vertical bars. Ordinate: contraction height as a percentage of the maximum response. Abscissa: final bath concentration (M) of dopamine on a log scale.[8] (Reprinted with permission of Br. J. Pharmacol.)

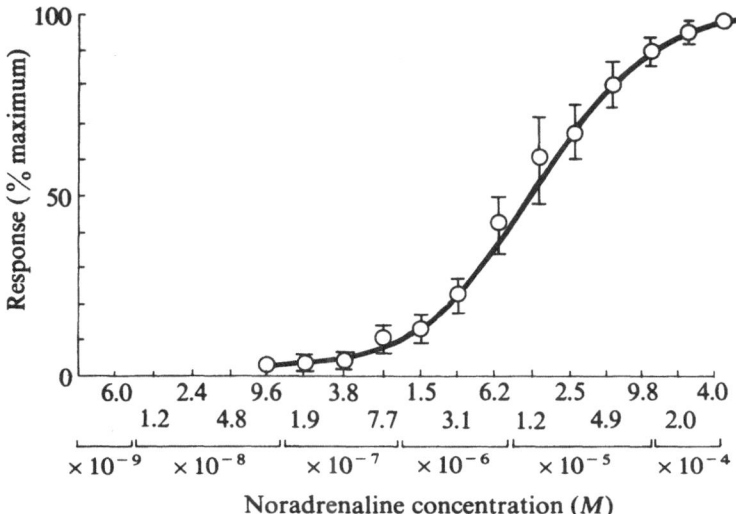

**Figure 6.20** Log concentration–response curve to $(-)$-noradrenaline for the mean response of the vasa deferentia from four rats. The vertical bars represent the standard errors of the means.[8] (Reprinted with permission of Br. J. Pharmacol.)

displaced to the right. The testes are then pushed into the abdominal cavity by the application of pressure to the scrotum. By lifting the terminal end of the colon the hypogastric nerves can be seen running along either side of the mesentary. While holding one testis the ductus deferens is freed from connective tissue and cut from the epididymis. The testis is then removed. By grasping the cut end of the ductus deferens it is separated from adjacent tissue.

One hypogastric nerve is tied and cut 5 cm from the ductus deferens. This piece is cleaned to within 0.5 cm of the organ. The remainder of the nerve up to the ductus is preserved by isolating the piece of peritoneum that contained it. The ductus deferens is then cut from the urethra and removed together with its nerve and the small piece of peritoneum and transferred to a bath consisting of Krebs solution. Dissection of the organ and the nerve is done in the solution. The contralateral side may be prepared in the same way.

The ductus deferens is tied by its proximal end to a glass rod and set up in an organ bath containing 12 ml of Krebs solution at 31°C which is aerated with a mixture of 95 % $O_2$ and 5 % $CO_2$. The distal end of the ductus is tied to a lever to which a 1 g load is suspended. The hypogastric nerve is passed through a channel of a pair of electrodes of the pattern described by Burn and Rand[17] and situated below the meniscus of the bath fluid. The preparation is electrically stimulated at a rate of 80/s using rectangular wave pulses of 2 ms duration for a period of 2 to 3 s. It is possible to use lower rates of stimulation applied for longer periods. The stimulus potential is usually 1 to 3 V. The nerve may be stimulated once every 2 min and will continue responding for several hours.

## Rat Fundus Strip

The rat fundus has been used extensively for in vitro experimentation concerned with the action of specific drugs and with revealing structure activity relations. In particular, this isolated preparation has been useful in experiments with serotonin (5-HT) and its antagonists, and it has largely replaced the rat uterus and guinea pig ileum in experimentation with 5-HT.[62] Cumulative dose-response data for 5-HT are readily attainable with the rat fundus strip. The selective sensitivity of the strip to 5-HT makes it a very suitable preparation for the assay of this substance in tissues and in biological fluids. Other (contaminating) substances in tissues and extracts are much less potent than 5-HT on the rat fundus. Indeed, it has been demonstrated that the only other substances that might interfere with the assay of 5-HT when this preparation is used are sympathomimetic amines. When their presence is suspected, they can be differentially destroyed.

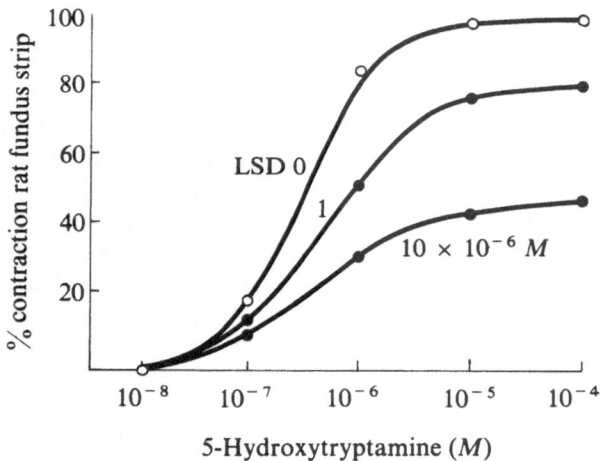

**Figure 6.21** Cumulative log concentration–response curves for 5-HT in the presence of various concentrations of LSD.[48] (Reprinted with permission of Arch. Int. Pharmacodyn.)

Offermeier and Ariëns[48] demonstrated that the serotonin-induced contraction of the fundus strip is most likely a direct action, in contrast to the probably indirect action of 5-HT on certain other muscle preparation (e.g., the calf tracheal muscle). Further, these investigators showed that the serotonin antagonists, LSD and methysergide, *do not* act competitively, as seen from the dose–response curves of Figures 6.21 and 6.22. It is of interest to note that certain agents sensitize the rat fundus to 5-HT. Among these sensitizers are imipramine and cocaine. The sensitizing action of cocaine is illustrated in Figure 6.23.

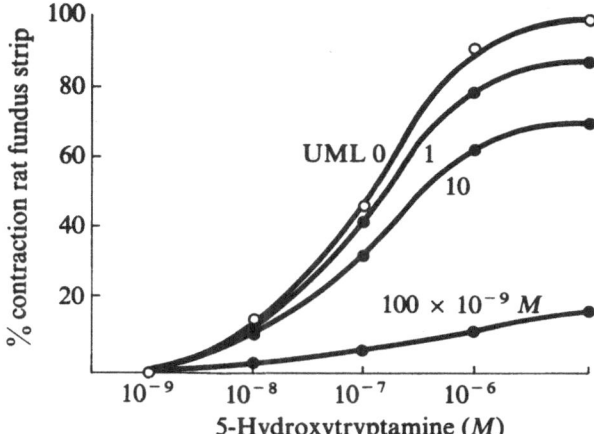

**Figure 6.22** Cumulative log concentration–response curves for 5-HT in the presence of various concentrations of methysergide (UML).[48] (Reprinted with permission of Arch. Int. Pharmacodyn.)

## Method of Preparation[62]

Rats of either sex are killed by a blow on the head. The abdomen is then opened. The entire stomach is dissected free from the abdomen and then placed into Krebs solution at 37°C and aerated with 95% $O_2$ and 5% $CO_2$. The fundal portion is recognized by its gray color; it is a translucent balloon-like tissue, capable of large changes in volume. The pyloric antrum, which is thicker and redder in color, is removed except for a band of pyloric tissue wide enough to

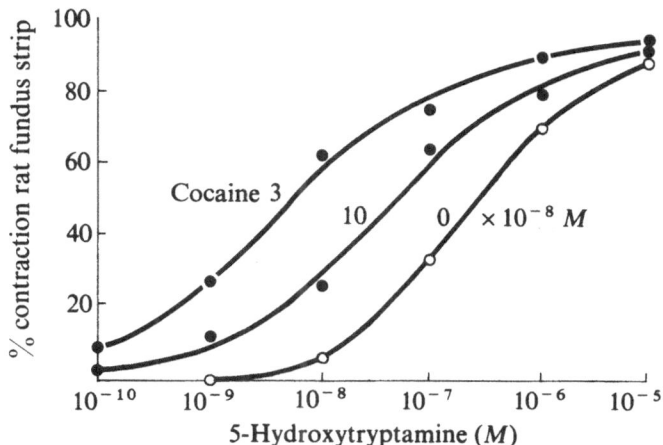

**Figure 6.23** Cumulative log concentration–response curves for 5-HT on the rat fundus strip in the presence of various concentrations of cocaine.[48] Cocaine sensitization at $3 \times 10^{-8}$ $M$ is greater than that at $10^{-7}$ $M$. (Reprinted with permission of Arch. Int. Pharmacodyn.)

be tied to a cannula. The fundal contents are washed away, the cannula tied into place, and the muscle suspended in a 40-ml organ bath at 37°C. The fundus is distended with 7 ml Krebs solution. The internal pressure can be recorded on a kymograph by a water manometer. The fundus is then taken off the cannula and cut into a strip, either by cutting spirally around the same plane as the circular muscle or by opening the fundus along the lesser curvature and cutting to preserve the longitudinal muscle. It is convenient to leave a small band of pyloric tissue attached to the fundus to act as a marker, and thus to prevent cutting in the wrong direction after the fundus has been opened into a flat plate. Cotton is then tied to the ends and the strip is gently stretched so that any protrusions and fringes of pyloric tissue may be trimmed away in order to give a long, clean, thin strip. One end of the strip is tied to the tissue holder and lowered into the organ bath. The cotton tied to the other end of the strip is attached to a recording lever. The preload is 1 g. The muscle does not relax spontaneously after contraction. It must be stretched to assist its recovery by adding an extra 1 g to the load. The preparation should be allowed to stretch for 30 min before use.


## Phrenic Nerve Diaphragm Preparation of the Rat

In 1946 Bülbring[14] described the phrenic nerve diaphragm preparation of the rat as a model for studying the effects of drugs on the twitches of diaphragm striated muscle in response to electrical stimulation of the phrenic nerve. It was thus being used as an isolated mammalian nerve–muscle preparation.

It was demonstrated that single submaximal shocks, when applied to the phrenic nerve, produced greater contractions of diaphragm muscle if epinephrine (50 mg) was added to the bath. This effect was observed whether epinephrine reached the site of nerve stimulation or not. Epinephrine had no effect on the muscle response to *maximal* nerve stimuli.

With slow rates of stimulation, muscle contraction elicited by maximal nerve stimuli was increased by the addition of small doses of eserine or prostigmine. Depression could be produced by prolonged drug action, by an overdose of the anticholinesterase, or by increasing the stimulation rate in the presence of the anticholinesterase. It was also observed that adrenaline could augment the action of eserine and prostigmine in this preparation. The size of the muscle contractions could be increased or decreased, depending on certain conditions. Muscle contractions were increased when the amount of the anticholinesterase was small and when the rate of stimulation was slow. The contractions were depressed by adrenaline after an overdose of the anticholinesterase or with faster rates of stimulation.

The depressant effect of eserine or prostigmine and the augmentation of this action by epinephrine are more readily observed in a fresh preparation than in one stimulated for several hours. The possibility that acetylcholine accumulated during the initial stages of motor nerve stimulation was raised.[14]

Atropine was found to have multiple effects. It increased only slightly the size of muscle contractions elicited by maximal nerve stimuli. However, if muscle contractions were increased by eserine or prostigmine, atropine reduced them to normal size. If muscle contractions were depressed by an overdose of an anticholinesterase or by a faster rate of stimulation, then atropine counteracted the depression.

In the presence of an anticholinesterase, it could be shown that curarine abolishes the depressant effects of excess acetylcholine. This effect occurs whether it is produced by rapid nerve stimulation or by adding acetylcholine to the bath. Atropine differed from curarine in that it abolished the depressant effect of rapid motor nerve stimulation but it did not abolish the depression caused by the addition of acetylcholine to the bath.

These observations, over 30 years ago, laid the foundation for the use of this preparation in the assay of neuromuscular blocking agents. Using this preparation one can show clearly the different effects of physostigmine and neostigmine on the neuromuscular block produced by "curarine-like" agents. Also, the increased effect of acetylcholine is demonstrated simply by blocking the destructive cholinesterases.

Using basic receptor terminology we designate the "skeletal muscle end plate receptor" which interacts with the endogenous neurotransmitter acetylcholine as the "nictotinic II receptor." It is now well known[64] that curarine-type agents act as competitive blockers of acetylcholine at this receptor in contrast to the succinylcholine-type agents that act as hyperdepolarizing blockers.

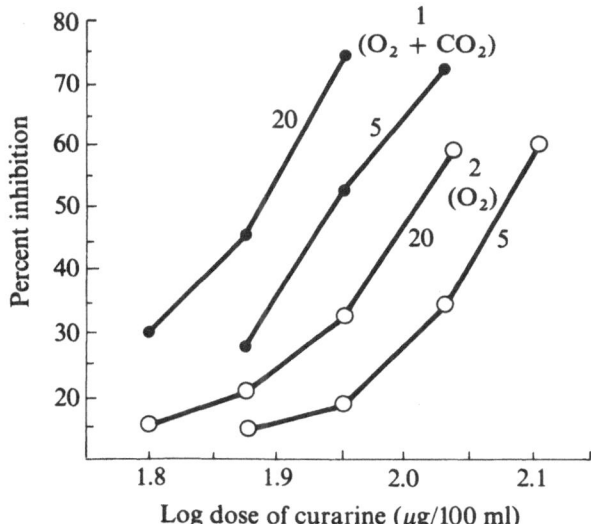

**Figure 6.24** Isolated phrenic nerve diaphragm of the rat. Abscissae: logarithm of tubocurarine concentration. Ordinates: percentage inhibition of muscle contractions. The effect of different rates of stimulation (20 and 5 min) on the action of tubocurarine is shown in two experiments (1 and 2).[19] (Reprinted with permission of Br. J. Pharmacol.)

Thus, in the latter group, duration of action will not be altered by using cholinesterase inhibitors.

Chou,[19] using the phrenic nerve diaphragm of the rat, demonstrated the relation between the logarithm of the concentration of tubocurarine and the percentage inhibition of muscle contractions (Fig. 6.24). It is evident that the effect produced by tubocurarine is greater when the muscle is working (higher stimulation rate). A variation in the strength of stimuli had no influence on the action of tubocurarine.

This preparation can be used to demonstate the clinical observations that certain antibiotics, e.g., neomycin and gentamicin, prolong the action of curarine-like agents. Brazil and Prado-Franceschi[10,11] investigated the action of neomycin and gentamicin on acetylcholine output. They found that both antibiotics drastically reduced the amount of acetylcholine released by motor nerve impulses. This is seen in Figures 6.25 and 6.26. Both antibiotics produced a shift to the right of the dose–response curve for acetylcholine. A (small) component of this action of the antibiotics is due to their antagonism of acetylcholine action on the muscle.

### Method of Preparation[14]

An adult rat is killed by a blow to the head and bled out so that the thorax is free of blood. The fur and skin are removed over the thorax and the thorax is opened along the right side of the sternum. The frontal part of the right thoracic

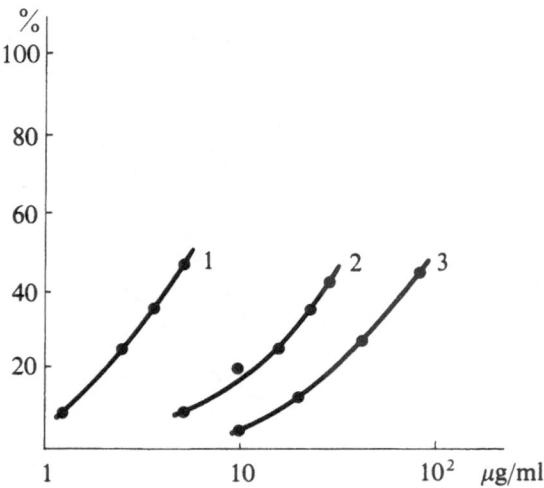

**Figure 6.25** Isolated denervated hemidiaphragm of the rat. Log dose–response curves for acetylcholine obtained in plain Tyrode solution and in the same solution containing two doses of neomycin (310 μg/ml and 620 μg/ml). (Reprinted with permission of Arch. Int. Pharmacodyn.)

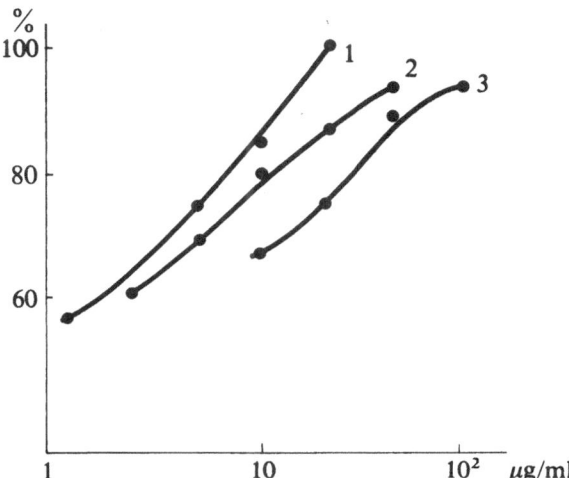

**Figure 6.26** Isolated denervated hemidiaphragm of the rat. Log dose–response curves for acetylcholine obtained in plain Tyrode solution and in the same solution containing two doses of gentamicin (608 μg/ml and 1216 μg/ml).[11] (Reprinted with permission Arch. Int. Pharmacodyn.)

wall is then removed. The mediastinum behind the sternum is severed, and a cut is made just above the frontal insertion of the diaphragm. The phrenic nerve sometimes attaches itself to the ribs and care must be taken so that damage does not occur. The frontal part of the thoracic wall is then removed, and the phrenic nerve is seen. Both left lobes of the lung are removed. The left abdominal muscles are cut along the costal margin and the last rib is held with a pair of forceps. A strip of diaphragm is now cut out. Two converging cuts are made through the ribs towards the tendinous part of the diaphragm parallel to its muscle fibers, 3 mm to the right and 3 mm to the left of the point where the phrenic nerve enters the diaphragm. The strip is cut out beyond the tendinous part with 2.5 cm of phrenic nerve attached to it. The preparation has a fan-like shape, being 3 mm wide at the tendinous end and 12 mm wide at the costal margin.

A thread is attached to the tendinous part while a second thread is attached to the cut end of the nerve. The preparation can be lifted by the thread attached to the diaphragm. It is lowered partly into an organ bath and the thread from the muscle is attached to an isotonic lever while that from the nerve is threaded through the electrode. The nerve is now drawn gently into the electrode. Krebs solution is used and is aerated with 95% $O_2$ and 5% $CO_2$ at a temperature of 37°C. The nerve is stimulated at 12 shocks per minute by rectangular wave pulses of 0.5 ms duration. The bath can be 50 ml and should be filled to the level of the upper electrode. In testing neuromuscular blockade the drug will usually produce its effect in 3 min; however, 6 to 10 min should be allowed for recovery after the drug has been washed out.

## Rat Uterus Preparation

Ahlquist[1] originally classified the rat uterus as a tissue possessing primarily $\beta$-adrenergic receptors. He based his conclusion on the observation that the order of potency of the adrenergic amines used was of the type which he ascribed to $\beta$-receptors in general. Ahlquist[2] also postulated that all uteri contain both $\alpha$-excitatory and $\beta$-inhibitory receptors. In 1962 Rudzik and Miller[54] reported that the uterine *inhibitory* responses to epinephrine, levarterenol, and phenylephrine could be prevented by the $\alpha$-adrenergic blocker phentolamine. In addition these uterine inhibitory responses could be blocked by the $\alpha$- and $\beta$-adrenergic receptor blocking agent dihydroergotamine. They reported the inhibitory response to isoproterenol could be blocked by dihydroergotamine. On the basis of this finding, Rudzik and Miller concluded that the rat uterus contained both $\alpha$- and $\beta$-receptors and that both receptors could produce relaxation or inhibition.

Levy and Tozzi[43] presented work challenging the concept that both $\alpha$- and $\beta$-receptors could produce relaxation in the rat uterus. They demonstrated that epinephrine, isoproprenol, and phenylephrine all produced uterine inhibitory responses that were not modified by $\alpha$-adrenergic blocking agents such as phentolamine, phenoxybenzamine, and tolazoline (Fig. 6.27). The uterine inhibitory responses to epinephrine, isoproterenol, and phenylephrine were blocked by all compounds possessing some degree of $\beta$-blocking activity. Thus, they were able to demonstrate the presence of only $\beta$-inhibitory receptors in isolated rat uterine segments.

By the late 1960s it was determined that stimulation of $\beta$-receptors by catecholamines caused an increase of cyclic adenosine 3′,5′-monophosphate (cAMP) levels in various tissues, including the rat uterus.

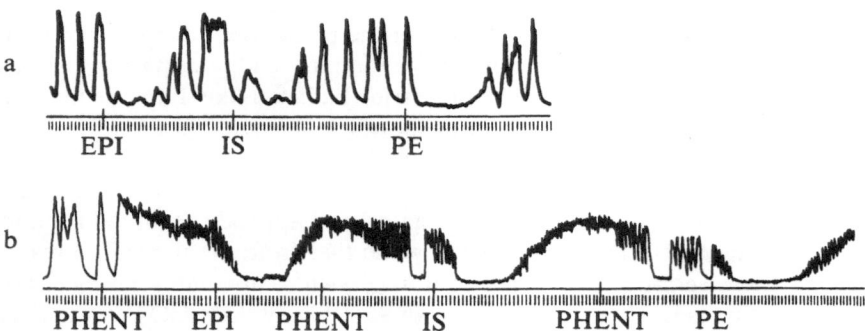

**Figure 6.27** The effects of epinephrine (EPI), isoproterenol (IS), and phenylephrine (PE) on isometric contractions of the isolated rat uterus are shown in the two panels. Panel a— control responses to EPI (0.01 $\mu$g/ml), IS (0.01 $\mu$g/ml), and PE (1 $\mu$g/ml). Panel b— responses to EPI, IS, and PE after phentolamine (PHENT) at a concentration of 50 $\mu$g/ml.[43] (Reprinted with permission of J. Pharmacol. Exp. Therap.)

Polacek and Daniel[44] confirmed the observation that adrenaline brings about relaxation of the isolated rat uterus and that this effect is accompanied by a marked increase of the cAMP level. They also showed that both mechanical and biochemical effects were $\beta$ responses because they were preserved in phenoxybenzamine-pretreated tissues and could be induced by the pure $\beta$ agent is oproterenol. These results provided some evidence for the conclusion that an increased intracellular concentration of cAMP can be related to the mechanical response of uterine relaxation. It is of interest that theophylline, a phosphodiesterase inhibitor, potentiates the relaxing effect of norepinephrine on the isolated uterus.

Historically this preparation is important because of its sensitivity to epinephrine and its relative insensitivity to norepinephrine. It should be noted, however, that it is remarkably sensitive to cholinergic agents, i.e., acetyl $\beta$-methylcholine[49] and the uterotonic stimulant oxytocin[53] (Fig. 6.28).

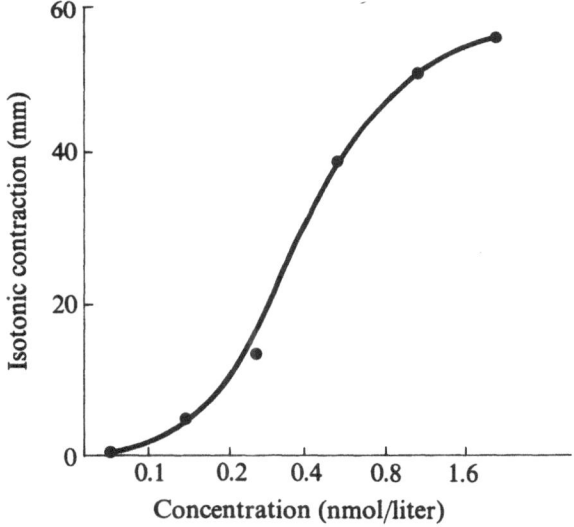

**Figure 6.28** Responses of the isolated rat uterus to cumulative doses of oxytocin. Ordinate represents isotonic contraction in millimeters of shortening and the abscissa is drug concentration in nanomoles per liter.[53] (Reprinted with permission of Eur. J. Pharmacol.)

## Method of Preparation

DeJalon and co-workers[35] in 1945 described the rat uterus preparation. A modified version follows:

Rats weighing 200–300 g are primed with doses of 10 $\mu$g/100 g of diethylstilbestrol given 24 hr prior to testing. The animal is then killed by a blow to the head and the abdomen opened. The intestine is pulled to the side and the two horns of the uterus are exposed. Mesenteric attachments are cut away and the two horns are placed in Locke solution. The horns are trimmed of fat and then each is cut open longitudinally. Each muscle segment may then be sub-divided. A thread is attached at each end and the uterine segment is suspended in a 10-ml volume, constant-temperature (37°C) bath containing Locke solution which is aerated with 95% $O_2$ and 5% $CO_2$. Spontaneous activity may be recorded isometrically by means of a force displacement transducer recording through a multichannel cathode ray tube camera system. A preload of 0.5 g is used. The preparation will take 30 min to "settle down" before regular responses are obtained.

Several points should be made about this preparation. First, when the drug is administered there is often a latent period before a response is seen. Second, the tissue will relax while the drug is still present; thus, the response is often not sustained. Finally, the maximum response is usually seen within 0.5 min.

## Frog Rectus Abdominus

This skeletal muscle preparation has been used extensively in order to study the physiology and pharmacology of the neuromuscular junction. Although this muscle is striated, its response to acetylcholine is a slow contraction. Langley[41] described this pharmacological response as a "protracted contraction for many minutes." It is believed that this type of response is due to the presence of a distinct, slow muscle fiber system which is innervated by small nerve fibers.[38] Forester and Schmidt,[25] using microelectrodes in the muscle, recorded the junctional potentials. They stimulated large and small nerve fibers and could distinguish two different groups of muscle fibers in the rectus. One group, located only at the ventral surface, were innervated by small (high-threshold) nerve fibers and produced typically small-nerve junction potentials. The other group, innervated only by large (low-threshold) nerve fibers, produced larger junction potentials. The membrane time-constant and input resistance of these fibers were similar to those of twitch fibers in other frog muscles. It was concluded that the rectus muscle, and other frog muscles, contained two distinct type of muscle fibers: twitch and slow.

Clark[20] demonstrated that the response of this preparation to acetycholine was greater with isotonic rather than isometric recording (Fig. 6.29).

Many other compounds are capable of contracting the frog rectus. Carbachol, butyrylcholine, and suxamethonium are examples. A dose–response curve for suxamethonium is shown in Figure 6.30.[12]

The action of acetylcholine on this preparation is antagonized competitively by $d$-tubocurarine, an antagonism similar to that seen in man. For example, a concentration of $2 \times 10^{-6}$ $M$ acetylcholine, which yields a contraction that is about 30% $E_{max}$, is almost completely abolished by $10^{-6}$ $M$ $d$-tubocurarine.[22] Gallamine ($10^{-4}$–$10^{-5}$ $M$) is also an effective competitive blocker of this

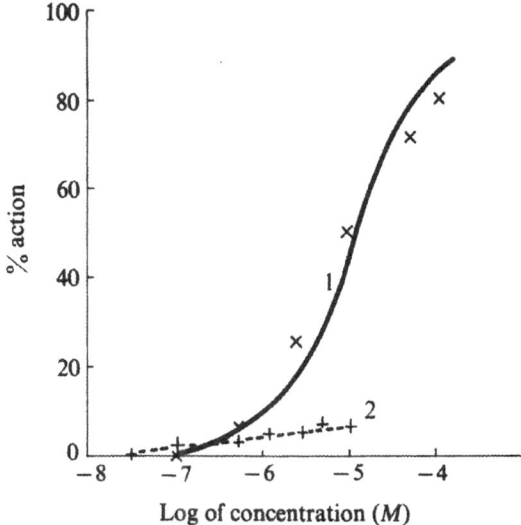

**Figure 6.29** Action of acetylcholine on the frog rectus abdominus. Curve 1, isotonic; curve 2, isometric.[20] (Reprinted with permission of J. Physiol.)

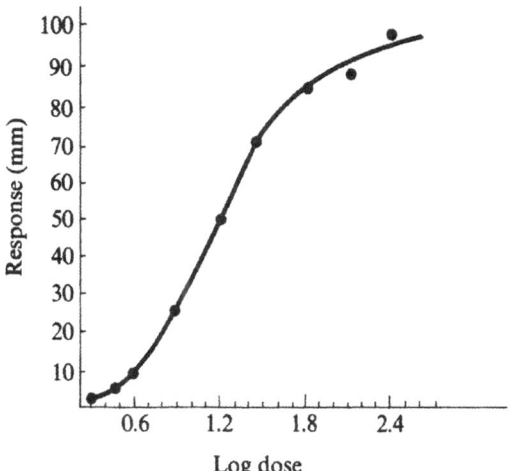

**Figure 6.30** Dose–response curve for suxamethonium using the frog rectus abdominus muscle. Abscissa, log dose in micrograms of suxamethonium in a 10-ml bath.[12] (Reprinted with permission of Brit. J. Pharmacol.)

concentration of acetylcholine in this preparation. Other agonists, such as suxamethonium and butyrylcholine, may be used to illustrate the blocking action of *d*-tubocurarine.

It is well known clinically that certain aminogylycosides block the myoneural junction of skeletal muscle. Jindal and Deshpande[36] used the frog rectus abdomenus to show the effect of streptomycin on acetylcholine-induced contractions. Doses of from 5 to 20 mg/ml could inhibit contraction to varying degrees. For example, 5 mg/ml of streptomycin reduced the effect of 1 mg/ml of acetylcholine by 37%, and a 46% reduction was produced with 20 mg/ml of streptomycin. These findings support the view that streptomycin, even in ordinary therapeutic doses, may produce some degree of neuromuscular blockade in some patients, thus confirming the observations of Loder and Walker.[45] Neostigmine and calcium ions are somewhat effective in overcoming the streptomycin inhibition.

### Method of Preparation[34]

A frog weighing about 20 g and of the species *Rana pipiens* is used, although Brittain et al.[12] used *Rana temporania*. The frog is pithed and then decapitated, destroying the spinal cord. The frog is placed on a dissecting board and its limbs are pinned down. The skin of the abdomen is lifted with forceps and is cut from above the sternum longitudinally downward across the abdomen. Lateral cuts are made to expose the entire abdomen. The two rectus muscles are seen running on each side of the midline from the base of the sternum downward. The muscles are then dissected free and transferred to Ringer's solution at room temperature. The muscles are subsequently divided longitudinally and a thread is attached to the top and bottom of each piece. The muscle is then suspended in a 10 ml organ bath with one thread attached to the base of the bath and other to the lever. The load on the lever is about 1 g. The bath fluid is oxygenated Ringer solution that is kept at room temperature.

It should be noted that after the muscle contracts it does not relax rapidly when the drug is washed out. To promote a more rapid relaxation the muscle may be stretched by gently increasing the load.

It is recommended that the preparation be stretched before experimentation with a 1 g preload for 30 min.

## Isolated Rabbit Heart

The isolated rabbit heart preparation is well suited for studies of cardiac drug action and, in particular, for studies involving autonomic stimulating and blocking drugs since it contains both $\beta$-adrenergic and muscarinic cholinergic receptors. In fact, the use of this preparation by Ahlquist[1] figures prominently in the classification of adrenoreceptors into the two classes, $\alpha$ and $\beta$. Ahlquist observed that epinephrine and norepinephrine increased both the rate and the amplitude of contractions in the isolated rabbit heart and, further, that these effects were accompanied by a concomitant decrease in coronary blood flow. These findings, coupled to other studies on noncardiac tissues, led to the ranking of potencies of adrenergic agents that act on the $\beta$-receptor: isoproterenol > epinephrine > norepinephrine, the order obtained in the heart through stimulation of these receptors. Although $\beta$ stimulation in the heart is excitatory, in noncardiac tissues these receptors are generally inhibitory. Excitatory adrenergic stimulation in noncardiac tissues is mediated through $\alpha$-receptors. In this class the potency order is norepinephrine > epinephrine > isoproterenol.[3] The classification into $\alpha$ and $\beta$ was sharpened by the finding of specific blocking drugs for each class (see also Chap. 1).

Since the cardiac adrenoreceptors are $\beta$, this preparation can be used to demonstrate both $\beta$-agonistic and $\beta$-antagonistic drug actions. In addition, one may observe in this preparation the cardiac effects of acetylcholine, which include hyperpolarization of the pacemaker membrane and the corresponding reduction in heart rate. The cardiac effects of acetylcholine are antagonized by atropine and are, therefore, muscarinic cholinergic receptors. These cholinergic responses are intensified by inhibitors of the cholinesterases. It is noteworthy that while the sinoatrial and atrioventricular nodes are quite sensitive to acetylcholine, the spontaneous activity in the bundle of His and the Purkinje system is relatively resistant to this agent. Acetylcholine has no obvious inotropic or chronotropic action on the ventricle.

Table 6.1 and Figure 6.31 are from Ahlquist's 1948 paper in which he discussed this preparation.[1]

**Table 6.1**
Comparative effects of the amines on the perfused rabbit heart[a]

| Amine | Increase in rate and amplitude (%) | | | Coronary flow (%) | |
|---|---|---|---|---|---|
| | $R - 1$[b] | $A - 1$[b] | $R - 2$[c] | D.F.[d] | I.F.[e] |
| Isoproterenol | 101 | 90 | 49 | 11 | 18 |
| Epinephrine | 75 | 70 | 26 | 11 | 15 |
| Norepinephrine | 38 | 35 | 0 | 20 | 3 |

[a] Averages obtained from 20 hearts in which each amine was tested in each heart in a dosage of 0.1 cc. M/10,000 solution injected into the coronary inflow. (From Ahlquist[1] with permission of Am. J. Physiol.)
[b] Increase in rate and amplitude at the time of maximum effect.
[c] Increase in rate about 2 min after injection.
[d] Decreased coronary inflow measured at point of maximum decrease.
[e] Increased coronary inflow measured at point of maximum increase.

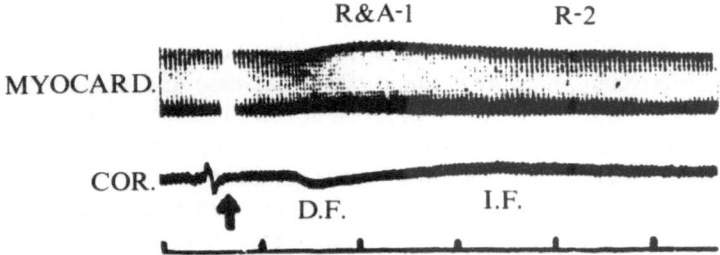

**Figure 6.31** Example of the action of the amines on the perfused rabbit heart. Cardiac contractions (myocard.) recorded with an optical lever. Coronary inflow (cor.) recorded with a rotameter. Time marks at 30-s intervals. The measurements listed in Table 6.1 were made at the indicated points: R & A-1, the increased rate and amplitude at the point of maximal effect; R-2, the increased rate at a point about 2 min after the amine administration (a measure of the duration of action); D.F., the decreased coronary inflow due to the increased myocardial activity; and I.F., the increased coronary flow due to the direct action on the coronary vessels. The amines were injected into the coronary inflow.[6] (Reprinted with permission of Am. J. Physiol.)

## Method of Preparation (Langendorff[40])

A rabbit is injected with 1000 U of heparin via the ear vein in order to inhibit subsequent clot formation. The animal is then killed by a blow to the head. The heart, along with 2–3 cm of attached aorta, is removed as quickly as possible. The preparation is then placed in oxygenated Locke solution for further preparation and dissection. In order to remove accumulated blood the preparation should be squeezed several times. The aorta is dissected free, and all of the other connecting vessels are carefully trimmed off. The aorta should be cut just below the point where it divides. The heart is then transferred to the perfusion apparatus, and the aorta is tied onto a glass cannula. Oxygenated Locke solution warmed to 37°C is applied from a reservoir maintained at a constant pressure. The pressure of the perfusing fluid keeps the aortic valve closed, thus allowing the fluid to pass through the coronary vessels and to exit from the inferior vena cava. A funnel is used to collect the fluid which exits. Flow can be measured instantaneously with a volume recorder.

Threads are attached to the ventricle by using a small hook which pierces the muscle. Threads are attached to the auricle by utilizing a small clip for attachment. These threads are connected to spring levers in order to record the size of the contractions.

Recordings of the coronary flow and of rate should be taken over 30-s intervals. Drugs are added to the cannula which enters the aorta and which contains the perfusing fluid. Responses usually occur in about 15 s and the effects last for several minutes. A 2-min period should lapse between dosing.

# References

1. Ahlquist, R. P.: Amer. J. Physiol., *153*:586, 1948.
2. Ahlquist, R. P.: Arch. Int. Pharmacodyn., *139*:38, 1962.
3. Ahlquist, R. P.: Ann. N.Y. Acad. Sci., *139*:549, 1967.
4. Akubue, P. I.: Br. J. Pharmacol., *27*:347, 1966.
5. Barlow, R. B., and Khan, I.: Br. J. Pharmacol., *14*:553, 1959.
6. Bennettt, A., Eley, K. G., and Scholes, G. B.: Br. J. Pharmacol., *34*:639, 1968.
7. Bergmann, F., Chaimovitz, M., and Wind, E.: Br. J. Pharmacol., *18*:381, 1962.
8. Birmingham, A. T., Paterson, G., and Wojcicki, J.: Br. J. Pharmacol., *39*:748, 1970.
9. Bohr, D. F.: Circ. Res., *32*:665, 1973.
10. Brazil, O. V., and Prado-Franceschi, J.: Arch. Int. Pharmacodyn., *179*:65, 1969.
11. Brazil, O. V., and Prado-Franceschi, J.: Arch. Int. Pharmacodyn., *179*:78, 1969.
12. Brittain, R. T., Chesher, B. G., Collier, H. O. J., and Grimshaw, J. J.: Br. J. Pharmacol., *14*:158, 1959.
13. Bülbring, E.: J. Physiol. (London), *125*:302, 1954.
14. Bülbring, E.: Br. J. Pharmacol., *1*:38, 1946.
15. Bülbring, E.: J. Physiol. (London), *128*:200, 1955.
16. Burgen, A. S. V., and Spero, L.: Br. J. Pharmacol., *40*:492, 1970.
17. Burn, J. H., and Rand, M. J.: J. Physiol. (London), *150*:295, 1960.
18. Burnstock, G., Holman, M. E., and Prosser, C. L.: Physiol. Rev., *43*:482, 1963.
19. Chou, T. C.: Br. J. Pharmacol., *2*:1, 1947.
20. Clark, A. J.: J. Physiol., *61*:530, 1926.
21. Cox, B. M., and Weinstock, M.: Br. J. Pharmacol., *27*:81, 1966.
22. Department of Pharmacology, University of Edinburgh: *Pharmacological Experiments on Isolated Preparations.* London, E. and S. Livingstone, 1970.
23. Emmelin, N., and MacIntosh, F. C.: J. Physiol. London, *131*:447, 1956.
24. Feldberg, W., and Gaddum, J. H.: J. Physiol. London, *81*:305, 1934.
25. Forrester, T., and Schmidt, H.: J. Physiol., *207*:477, 1970.
26. Furchgott, R. F.: Pharm. Rev., *7*:183, 1955.
27. Furchgott, R. F.: Ann. Rev. Pharm., *4*:21, 1964.
28. Furchgott, R. F.. and Bhadrakom, S.: J. Pharmacol. Exp. Ther., *108*: 129, 1953.
29. Furchgott, R. F.: In *Methods in Medical Research,* Vol. 8. (H. D. Bruner, ed.) Chicago, Year Book, 1960, pp 177–186.
30. Gero, A.: Mol. Pharmacol., *1*:312, 1965.
31. Gero, A., and Gurland, S.: Arch. Int. Pharmacodyn., *183*:25, 1970.
32. Hukovic, S.: Br. J. Pharmacol., *16*:188, 1961.
33. Jacob, L. S., and Tallarida, R. J.: Arch. Int. Pharmacodyn., *225*:166, 1977.
34. de Jalon, P. D. G.: Quart. J. Pharmacol., *20*:28, 1947.
35. de Jalon, P. D. G., Bayo, A., and de Jalon, P.: Farmacoter. Act., *3*:313, 1945.
36. Jindal, M. N., and Deshpande, V. R.: Br. J. Pharmacol., *15*:506, 1960.
37. Koelle, G. B.: In *The Pharmacological Basis of Therapeutics,* 5th ed. (Goodman and Gilman, eds.), New York, MacMillan, 1975, pp. 468.
38. Kuffler, S. W., and Williams, E. M. V.: J. Physiol., *121*:318, 1953.
39. Lands, A. M.: Pharm. Rev., *1*:279, 1949.
40. Langendorff, O.: Arch. für die gesamte Physiol., *61*:291, 1895.
41. Langley, J. N.: J. Physiol. *47*:159, 1913.
42. Leach, G. D.: J. Pharm. Pharmacol., *8*:501, 1956.
43. Levy, B., and Tozzi, S.: J. Pharmacol. Exp. Therap., *142*:178, 1963.
44. Levy, B., and Wilkenfeld, B. E.: Br. J. Pharmacol., *34*:604, 1968.
45. Loder, R. E.. and Walker, G. F.: Lancet, *2*:1812, 1959.

46. MacNab, M. W. Ph.D. Thesis, Temple University Medical School, Philadelphia, Pa., 1974.
47. Magnus, R.: Pflug. Arch. Ges. Physiol., *102*:349, 1904.
48. Offermeier, J., and Ariens, E. J.: Arch. Int. Pharmacodyn., *164*:192, 1966.
49. Olsson, O. A., and Persson, C. G. A.: J. Pharm. Pharmacol., *23*:878, 1971.
50. Paton, W. D. M.: J. Physiol., *127*:40P, 1955.
51. Paton, W. D. M.: Br. J. Pharmacol., *12*:119, 1957.
52. Polacek, I., and Daniel, E. E.: Can. J. Physiol. Pharmacol., *49*:988, 1971.
53. Polacek, I., Krejci, I., Nesvadba, H., and Rudinger: J. Eur. J. Pharmacol., *9*:239, 1970.
54. Rudzik, A. D., and Miller, J. W.: J. Pharmacol. Exp. Therap., *138*:82, 1962.
55. Sanner, J. H.: Arch. Int. Pharmacodyn., *180*: 46, 1969.
56. Schaumann, W.: Path. Pharmak., *223*:112, 1958.
57. Seferna, I., Loukomskaya, N., Kadlec, O., *et al*: J. Pharm. Pharmacol., *18*:501, 1966.
58. Somlyo, A. P., and Somlyo, A. V.: Pharm. Rev., *20*:197, 1968.
59. Somlyo, A. P., and Somlyo, A. V.: Pharm. Rev., *22*:249, 1970.
60. Tallarida, R. J., Sevy, R. W., Harakal, C., and Loughnane, M.: IEEE Trans, Biomed. Eng., *22*: 493, 1975.
61. Van Den Brink, F. G., and Lien, E. J.: Eur. J. Pharmacol., *44*:251, 1977.
62. Vane, J. R.: Br. J. Pharmacol., *12*:344, 1957.
63. Volle, R. L.: In *Drill's Pharmacology In Medicine* 4th ed. (J. R. DiPalma, ed.) New York, McGraw-Hill, 1971, pp. 584.
64. Waud, D. R. and Waud, B. E. in *Drill's Pharmacology in Medicine* 4th ed., J. R. DiPalma, ed.) McGraw-Hill, 1971, Chap. 36.

# Mathematical Tables

**Table A.1**
Areas under the standard normal curve

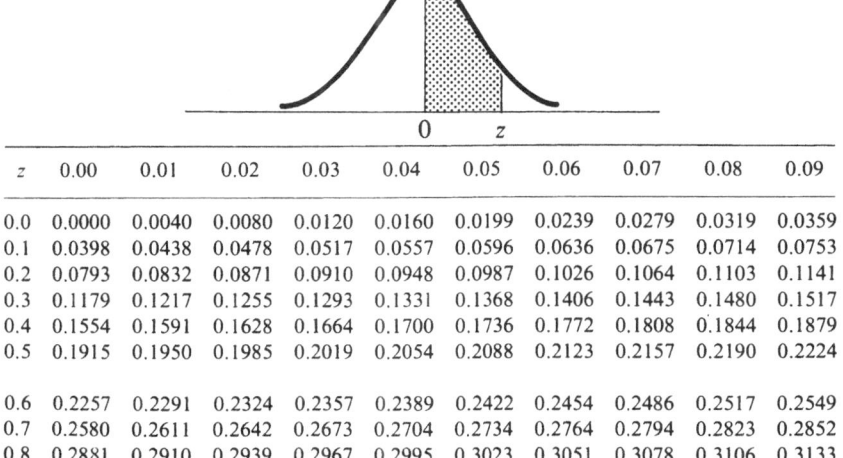

| $z$ | 0.00 | 0.01 | 0.02 | 0.03 | 0.04 | 0.05 | 0.06 | 0.07 | 0.08 | 0.09 |
|---|---|---|---|---|---|---|---|---|---|---|
| 0.0 | 0.0000 | 0.0040 | 0.0080 | 0.0120 | 0.0160 | 0.0199 | 0.0239 | 0.0279 | 0.0319 | 0.0359 |
| 0.1 | 0.0398 | 0.0438 | 0.0478 | 0.0517 | 0.0557 | 0.0596 | 0.0636 | 0.0675 | 0.0714 | 0.0753 |
| 0.2 | 0.0793 | 0.0832 | 0.0871 | 0.0910 | 0.0948 | 0.0987 | 0.1026 | 0.1064 | 0.1103 | 0.1141 |
| 0.3 | 0.1179 | 0.1217 | 0.1255 | 0.1293 | 0.1331 | 0.1368 | 0.1406 | 0.1443 | 0.1480 | 0.1517 |
| 0.4 | 0.1554 | 0.1591 | 0.1628 | 0.1664 | 0.1700 | 0.1736 | 0.1772 | 0.1808 | 0.1844 | 0.1879 |
| 0.5 | 0.1915 | 0.1950 | 0.1985 | 0.2019 | 0.2054 | 0.2088 | 0.2123 | 0.2157 | 0.2190 | 0.2224 |
| 0.6 | 0.2257 | 0.2291 | 0.2324 | 0.2357 | 0.2389 | 0.2422 | 0.2454 | 0.2486 | 0.2517 | 0.2549 |
| 0.7 | 0.2580 | 0.2611 | 0.2642 | 0.2673 | 0.2704 | 0.2734 | 0.2764 | 0.2794 | 0.2823 | 0.2852 |
| 0.8 | 0.2881 | 0.2910 | 0.2939 | 0.2967 | 0.2995 | 0.3023 | 0.3051 | 0.3078 | 0.3106 | 0.3133 |
| 0.9 | 0.3159 | 0.3186 | 0.3212 | 0.3238 | 0.3264 | 0.3289 | 0.3315 | 0.3340 | 0.3365 | 0.3389 |
| 1.0 | 0.3413 | 0.3438 | 0.3461 | 0.3485 | 0.3508 | 0.3531 | 0.3554 | 0.3577 | 0.3599 | 0.3621 |

*(Continued)*

**Table A.1** (*Continued*)

| $z$ | 0.00 | 0.01 | 0.02 | 0.03 | 0.04 | 0.05 | 0.06 | 0.07 | 0.08 | 0.09 |
|-----|------|------|------|------|------|------|------|------|------|------|
| 1.1 | 0.3643 | 0.3665 | 0.3686 | 0.3708 | 0.3729 | 0.3749 | 0.3770 | 0.3790 | 0.3810 | 0.3830 |
| 1.2 | 0.3849 | 0.3869 | 0.3888 | 0.3907 | 0.3925 | 0.3944 | 0.3962 | 0.3980 | 0.3997 | 0.4015 |
| 1.3 | 0.4032 | 0.4049 | 0.4066 | 0.4082 | 0.4099 | 0.4115 | 0.4131 | 0.4147 | 0.4162 | 0.4177 |
| 1.4 | 0.4192 | 0.4207 | 0.4222 | 0.4236 | 0.4251 | 0.4265 | 0.4279 | 0.4292 | 0.4306 | 0.4319 |
| 1.5 | 0.4332 | 0.4345 | 0.4357 | 0.4370 | 0.4382 | 0.4394 | 0.4406 | 0.4418 | 0.4429 | 0.4441 |
| 1.6 | 0.4452 | 0.4463 | 0.4474 | 0.4484 | 0.4495 | 0.4505 | 0.4515 | 0.4525 | 0.4535 | 0.4545 |
| 1.7 | 0.4554 | 0.4564 | 0.4573 | 0.4582 | 0.4591 | 0.4599 | 0.4608 | 0.4616 | 0.4625 | 0.4633 |
| 1.8 | 0.4641 | 0.4649 | 0.4656 | 0.4664 | 0.4671 | 0.4678 | 0.4686 | 0.4693 | 0.4699 | 0.4706 |
| 1.9 | 0.4713 | 0.4719 | 0.4726 | 0.4732 | 0.4738 | 0.4744 | 0.4750 | 0.4756 | 0.4761 | 0.4767 |
| 2.0 | 0.4772 | 0.4778 | 0.4783 | 0.4788 | 0.4793 | 0.4798 | 0.4803 | 0.4808 | 0.4812 | 0.4817 |
| 2.1 | 0.4821 | 0.4826 | 0.4830 | 0.4834 | 0.4838 | 0.4842 | 0.4846 | 0.4850 | 0.4854 | 0.4857 |
| 2.2 | 0.4861 | 0.4864 | 0.4868 | 0.4871 | 0.4875 | 0.4878 | 0.4881 | 0.4884 | 0.4887 | 0.4890 |
| 2.3 | 0.4893 | 0.4896 | 0.4898 | 0.4901 | 0.4904 | 0.4906 | 0.4909 | 0.4911 | 0.4913 | 0.4916 |
| 2.4 | 0.4918 | 0.4920 | 0.4922 | 0.4925 | 0.4927 | 0.4929 | 0.4931 | 0.4932 | 0.4934 | 0.4936 |
| 2.5 | 0.4938 | 0.4940 | 0.4941 | 0.4943 | 0.4945 | 0.4946 | 0.4948 | 0.4949 | 0.4951 | 0.4952 |
| 2.6 | 0.4953 | 0.4955 | 0.4956 | 0.4957 | 0.4959 | 0.4960 | 0.4961 | 0.4962 | 0.4963 | 0.4964 |
| 2.7 | 0.4965 | 0.4966 | 0.4967 | 0.4968 | 0.4969 | 0.4970 | 0.4971 | 0.4972 | 0.4973 | 0.4974 |
| 2.8 | 0.4974 | 0.4975 | 0.4976 | 0.4977 | 0.4977 | 0.4978 | 0.4979 | 0.4979 | 0.4980 | 0.4981 |
| 2.9 | 0.4981 | 0.4982 | 0.4982 | 0.4983 | 0.4984 | 0.4984 | 0.4985 | 0.4985 | 0.4986 | 0.4986 |
| 3.0 | 0.4987 | 0.4987 | 0.4987 | 0.4988 | 0.4988 | 0.4989 | 0.4989 | 0.4989 | 0.4990 | 0.4990 |

**Table A.2**
$t$ Distribution

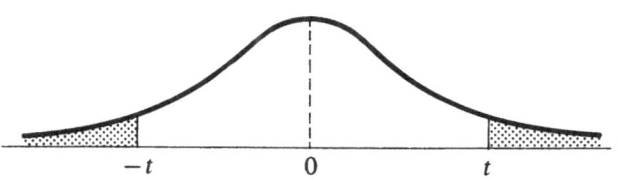

| deg. freedom, $v$ | 90% $(P = 0.1)$ | 95% $(P = 0.05)$ | 99% $(P = 0.01)$ |
|---|---|---|---|
| 1 | 6.314 | 12.706 | 63.657 |
| 2 | 2.920 | 4.303 | 9.925 |
| 3 | 2.353 | 3.182 | 5.841 |
| 4 | 2.132 | 2.776 | 4.604 |
| 5 | 2.015 | 2.571 | 4.032 |
| 6 | 1.943 | 2.447 | 3.707 |
| 7 | 1.895 | 2.365 | 3.499 |
| 8 | 1.860 | 2.306 | 3.355 |
| 9 | 1.833 | 2.262 | 3.250 |
| 10 | 1.812 | 2.228 | 3.169 |
| 11 | 1.796 | 2.201 | 3.106 |
| 12 | 1.782 | 2.179 | 3.055 |
| 13 | 1.771 | 2.160 | 3.012 |
| 14 | 1.761 | 2.145 | 2.977 |
| 15 | 1.753 | 2.131 | 2.947 |
| 16 | 1.746 | 2.120 | 2.921 |
| 17 | 1.740 | 2.110 | 2.898 |
| 18 | 1.734 | 2.101 | 2.878 |
| 19 | 1.729 | 2.093 | 2.861 |
| 20 | 1.725 | 2.086 | 2.845 |
| 21 | 1.721 | 2.080 | 2.831 |
| 22 | 1.717 | 2.074 | 2.819 |
| 23 | 1.714 | 2.069 | 2.807 |
| 24 | 1.711 | 2.064 | 2.797 |
| 25 | 1.708 | 2.060 | 2.787 |
| 26 | 1.706 | 2.056 | 2.779 |
| 27 | 1.703 | 2.052 | 2.771 |
| 28 | 1.701 | 2.048 | 2.763 |
| 29 | 1.699 | 2.045 | 2.756 |
| inf. | 1.645 | 1.960 | 2.576 |

**Table A.3**
Probit transformation[a]

| % | | % | | % | | % | | % | |
|---|---|---|---|---|---|---|---|---|---|
| 0 | | 20 | 4.1584 | 40 | 4.7467 | 60 | 5.2533 | 80 | 5.8416 |
| 1 | 2.6737 | 21 | 4.1936 | 41 | 4.7725 | 61 | 5.2793 | 81 | 5.8779 |
| 2 | 2.9463 | 22 | 4.2278 | 42 | 4.7981 | 62 | 5.3055 | 82 | 5.9154 |
| 3 | 3.1192 | 23 | 4.2612 | 43 | 4.8236 | 63 | 5.3319 | 83 | 5.9542 |
| 4 | 3.2493 | 24 | 4.2937 | 44 | 4.8490 | 64 | 5.3585 | 84 | 5.9945 |
| 5 | 3.3551 | 25 | 4.3255 | 45 | 4.8743 | 65 | 5.3853 | 85 | 6.0364 |
| 6 | 3.4452 | 26 | 4.3567 | 46 | 4.8996 | 66 | 5.4125 | 86 | 6.0803 |
| 7 | 3.5242 | 27 | 4.3872 | 47 | 4.9247 | 67 | 5.4399 | 87 | 6.1264 |
| 8 | 3.5949 | 28 | 4.4172 | 48 | 4.9498 | 68 | 5.4677 | 88 | 6.1750 |
| 9 | 3.6592 | 29 | 4.4466 | 49 | 4.9749 | 69 | 5.4959 | 89 | 6.2265 |
| 10 | 3.7184 | 30 | 4.4756 | 50 | 5.0000 | 70 | 5.5244 | 90 | 6.2816 |
| 11 | 3.7735 | 31 | 4.5041 | 51 | 5.0251 | 71 | 5.5534 | 91 | 6.3408 |
| 12 | 3.8250 | 32 | 4.5323 | 52 | 5.0502 | 72 | 5.5828 | 92 | 6.4051 |
| 13 | 3.8736 | 33 | 4.5601 | 53 | 5.0753 | 73 | 5.6128 | 93 | 6.4758 |
| 14 | 3.9197 | 34 | 4.5875 | 54 | 5.1004 | 74 | 5.6433 | 94 | 6.5548 |
| 15 | 3.9636 | 35 | 4.6147 | 55 | 5.1257 | 75 | 5.6745 | 95 | 6.6449 |
| 16 | 4.0055 | 36 | 4.6415 | 56 | 5.1510 | 76 | 5.7063 | 96 | 6.7507 |
| 17 | 4.0458 | 37 | 4.6681 | 57 | 5.1764 | 77 | 5.7388 | 97 | 6.8808 |
| 18 | 4.0846 | 38 | 4.6945 | 58 | 5.2019 | 78 | 5.7722 | 98 | 7.0537 |
| 19 | 4.1221 | 39 | 4.7207 | 59 | 5.2275 | 79 | 5.8064 | 99 | 7.3263 |

[a] The percentages of the area under the normal distribution curve from negative infinity and the corresponding probits.

**Table A.4**
Common logarithms

| n | 0 | 1 | 2 | 3 | 4 | 5 | 6 | 7 | 8 | 9 |
|---|---|---|---|---|---|---|---|---|---|---|
| 1.0 | 0.0000 | 0.0043 | 0.0086 | 0.0128 | 0.0170 | 0.0212 | 0.0253 | 0.0294 | 0.0334 | 0.0374 |
| 1.1 | 0.0414 | 0.0453 | 0.0492 | 0.0531 | 0.0569 | 0.0607 | 0.0645 | 0.0682 | 0.0719 | 0.0755 |
| 1.2 | 0.0792 | 0.0828 | 0.0864 | 0.0899 | 0.0934 | 0.0969 | 0.1004 | 0.1038 | 0.1072 | 0.1106 |
| 1.3 | 0.1139 | 0.1173 | 0.1206 | 0.1239 | 0.1271 | 0.1303 | 0.1335 | 0.1367 | 0.1399 | 0.1430 |
| 1.4 | 0.1461 | 0.1492 | 0.1523 | 0.1553 | 0.1584 | 0.1614 | 0.1644 | 0.1673 | 0.1703 | 0.1732 |
| 1.5 | 0.1761 | 0.1790 | 0.1818 | 0.1847 | 0.1875 | 0.1903 | 0.1931 | 0.1959 | 0.1987 | 0.2014 |
| 1.6 | 0.2041 | 0.2068 | 0.2095 | 0.2122 | 0.2148 | 0.2175 | 0.2201 | 0.2227 | 0.2253 | 0.2279 |
| 1.7 | 0.2304 | 0.2330 | 0.2355 | 0.2380 | 0.2405 | 0.2430 | 0.2455 | 0.2480 | 0.2504 | 0.2529 |
| 1.8 | 0.2553 | 0.2577 | 0.2601 | 0.2625 | 0.2648 | 0.2672 | 0.2695 | 0.2718 | 0.2742 | 0.2765 |
| 1.9 | 0.2788 | 0.2810 | 0.2833 | 0.2856 | 0.2878 | 0.2900 | 0.2923 | 0.2945 | 0.2967 | 0.2989 |
| 2.0 | 0.3010 | 0.3032 | 0.3054 | 0.3075 | 0.3096 | 0.3118 | 0.3139 | 0.3160 | 0.3181 | 0.3201 |
| 2.1 | 0.3222 | 0.3243 | 0.3263 | 0.3284 | 0.3304 | 0.3324 | 0.3345 | 0.3365 | 0.3385 | 0.3404 |
| 2.2 | 0.3424 | 0.3444 | 0.3464 | 0.3483 | 0.3502 | 0.3522 | 0.3541 | 0.3560 | 0.3579 | 0.3598 |
| 2.3 | 0.3617 | 0.3636 | 0.3655 | 0.3674 | 0.3692 | 0.3711 | 0.3729 | 0.3747 | 0.3766 | 0.3784 |
| 2.4 | 0.3802 | 0.3820 | 0.3838 | 0.3856 | 0.3874 | 0.3892 | 0.3909 | 0.3927 | 0.3945 | 0.3962 |
| 2.5 | 0.3979 | 0.3997 | 0.4014 | 0.4031 | 0.4048 | 0.4065 | 0.4082 | 0.4099 | 0.4116 | 0.4133 |
| 2.6 | 0.4150 | 0.4166 | 0.4183 | 0.4200 | 0.4216 | 0.4232 | 0.4249 | 0.4265 | 0.4281 | 0.4298 |
| 2.7 | 0.4314 | 0.4330 | 0.4346 | 0.4362 | 0.4378 | 0.4393 | 0.4409 | 0.4425 | 0.4440 | 0.4456 |
| 2.8 | 0.4472 | 0.4487 | 0.4502 | 0.4518 | 0.4533 | 0.4548 | 0.4564 | 0.4579 | 0.4594 | 0.4609 |
| 2.9 | 0.4624 | 0.4639 | 0.4654 | 0.4669 | 0.4683 | 0.4698 | 0.4713 | 0.4728 | 0.4742 | 0.4757 |
| 3.0 | 0.4771 | 0.4786 | 0.4800 | 0.4814 | 0.4829 | 0.4843 | 0.4857 | 0.4871 | 0.4886 | 0.4900 |
| 3.1 | 0.4914 | 0.4928 | 0.4942 | 0.4955 | 0.4969 | 0.4983 | 0.4997 | 0.5011 | 0.5024 | 0.5038 |
| 3.2 | 0.5051 | 0.5065 | 0.5079 | 0.5092 | 0.5105 | 0.5119 | 0.5132 | 0.5145 | 0.5159 | 0.5172 |
| 3.3 | 0.5185 | 0.5198 | 0.5211 | 0.5224 | 0.5237 | 0.5250 | 0.5263 | 0.5276 | 0.5289 | 0.5302 |
| 3.4 | 0.5315 | 0.5328 | 0.5340 | 0.5353 | 0.5366 | 0.5378 | 0.5391 | 0.5403 | 0.5416 | 0.5428 |
| 3.5 | 0.5441 | 0.5453 | 0.5465 | 0.5478 | 0.5490 | 0.5502 | 0.5514 | 0.5527 | 0.5539 | 0.5551 |
| 3.6 | 0.5563 | 0.5575 | 0.5587 | 0.5599 | 0.5611 | 0.5623 | 0.5635 | 0.5647 | 0.5658 | 0.5670 |
| 3.7 | 0.5682 | 0.5694 | 0.5705 | 0.5717 | 0.5729 | 0.5740 | 0.5752 | 0.5763 | 0.5775 | 0.5786 |
| 3.8 | 0.5798 | 0.5809 | 0.5821 | 0.5832 | 0.5843 | 0.5855 | 0.5866 | 0.5877 | 0.5888 | 0.5899 |
| 3.9 | 0.5911 | 0.5922 | 0.5933 | 0.5944 | 0.5955 | 0.5966 | 0.5977 | 0.5988 | 0.5999 | 0.6010 |
| 4.0 | 0.6021 | 0.6031 | 0.6042 | 0.6053 | 0.6064 | 0.6075 | 0.6085 | 0.6096 | 0.6107 | 0.6117 |
| 4.1 | 0.6128 | 0.6138 | 0.6149 | 0.6160 | 0.6170 | 0.6180 | 0.6191 | 0.6201 | 0.6212 | 0.6222 |
| 4.2 | 0.6232 | 0.6243 | 0.6253 | 0.6263 | 0.6274 | 0.6284 | 0.6294 | 0.6304 | 0.6314 | 0.6325 |
| 4.3 | 0.6335 | 0.6345 | 0.6355 | 0.6365 | 0.6375 | 0.6385 | 0.6395 | 0.6405 | 0.6415 | 0.6425 |
| 4.4 | 0.6435 | 0.6444 | 0.6454 | 0.6464 | 0.6474 | 0.6484 | 0.6493 | 0.6503 | 0.6513 | 0.6522 |
| 4.5 | 0.6532 | 0.6542 | 0.6551 | 0.6561 | 0.6571 | 0.6580 | 0.6590 | 0.6599 | 0.6609 | 0.6618 |
| 4.6 | 0.6628 | 0.6637 | 0.6646 | 0.6656 | 0.6665 | 0.6675 | 0.6684 | 0.6693 | 0.6702 | 0.6712 |
| 4.7 | 0.6721 | 0.6730 | 0.6739 | 0.6749 | 0.6758 | 0.6767 | 0.6776 | 0.6785 | 0.6794 | 0.6803 |
| 4.8 | 0.6812 | 0.6821 | 0.6830 | 0.6839 | 0.6848 | 0.6857 | 0.6866 | 0.6875 | 0.6884 | 0.6893 |
| 4.9 | 0.6902 | 0.6911 | 0.6920 | 0.6928 | 0.6937 | 0.6946 | 0.6955 | 0.6964 | 0.6972 | 0.6981 |

*(Continued)*

**Table A.4** (*Continued*)

| $n$ | 0 | 1 | 2 | 3 | 4 | 5 | 6 | 7 | 8 | 9 |
|-----|------|------|------|------|------|------|------|------|------|------|
| 5.0 | 0.6990 | 0.6998 | 0.7007 | 0.7016 | 0.7024 | 0.7033 | 0.7042 | 0.7050 | 0.7059 | 0.7067 |
| 5.1 | 0.7076 | 0.7084 | 0.7093 | 0.7101 | 0.7110 | 0.7118 | 0.7126 | 0.7135 | 0.7143 | 0.7152 |
| 5.2 | 0.7160 | 0.7168 | 0.7177 | 0.7185 | 0.7193 | 0.7202 | 0.7210 | 0.7218 | 0.7226 | 0.7235 |
| 5.3 | 0.7243 | 0.7251 | 0.7259 | 0.7267 | 0.7275 | 0.7284 | 0.7292 | 0.7300 | 0.7308 | 0.7316 |
| 5.4 | 0.7324 | 0.7332 | 0.7340 | 0.7348 | 0.7356 | 0.7364 | 0.7372 | 0.7380 | 0.7388 | 0.7396 |
| 5.5 | 0.7404 | 0.7412 | 0.7419 | 0.7427 | 0.7435 | 0.7443 | 0.7451 | 0.7459 | 0.7466 | 0.7474 |
| 5.6 | 0.7482 | 0.7490 | 0.7497 | 0.7505 | 0.7513 | 0.7520 | 0.7528 | 0.7536 | 0.7543 | 0.7551 |
| 5.7 | 0.7559 | 0.7566 | 0.7574 | 0.7582 | 0.7589 | 0.7597 | 0.7604 | 0.7612 | 0.7619 | 0.7627 |
| 5.8 | 0.7634 | 0.7642 | 0.7649 | 0.7657 | 0.7664 | 0.7672 | 0.7679 | 0.7686 | 0.7694 | 0.7701 |
| 5.9 | 0.7709 | 0.7716 | 0.7723 | 0.7731 | 0.7738 | 0.7745 | 0.7752 | 0.7760 | 0.7767 | 0.7774 |
| 6.0 | 0.7782 | 0.7789 | 0.7796 | 0.7803 | 0.7810 | 0.7818 | 0.7825 | 0.7832 | 0.7839 | 0.7846 |
| 6.1 | 0.7853 | 0.7860 | 0.7868 | 0.7875 | 0.7882 | 0.7889 | 0.7896 | 0.7903 | 0.7910 | 0.7917 |
| 6.2 | 0.7924 | 0.7931 | 0.7938 | 0.7945 | 0.7952 | 0.7959 | 0.7966 | 0.7973 | 0.7980 | 0.7987 |
| 6.3 | 0.7993 | 0.8000 | 0.8007 | 0.8014 | 0.8021 | 0.8028 | 0.8035 | 0.8041 | 0.8048 | 0.8055 |
| 6.4 | 0.8062 | 0.8069 | 0.8075 | 0.8082 | 0.8089 | 0.8096 | 0.8102 | 0.8109 | 0.8116 | 0.8122 |
| 6.5 | 0.8129 | 0.8136 | 0.8142 | 0.8149 | 0.8156 | 0.8162 | 0.8169 | 0.8176 | 0.8182 | 0.8189 |
| 6.6 | 0.8195 | 0.8202 | 0.8209 | 0.8215 | 0.8222 | 0.8228 | 0.8235 | 0.8241 | 0.8248 | 0.8254 |
| 6.7 | 0.8261 | 0.8267 | 0.8274 | 0.8280 | 0.8287 | 0.8293 | 0.8299 | 0.8306 | 0.8312 | 0.8319 |
| 6.8 | 0.8325 | 0.8331 | 0.8338 | 0.8344 | 0.8351 | 0.8357 | 0.8363 | 0.8370 | 0.8376 | 0.8382 |
| 6.9 | 0.8388 | 0.8395 | 0.8401 | 0.8407 | 0.8414 | 0.8420 | 0.8426 | 0.8432 | 0.8439 | 0.8445 |
| 7.0 | 0.8451 | 0.8457 | 0.8463 | 0.8470 | 0.8476 | 0.8482 | 0.8488 | 0.8494 | 0.8500 | 0.8506 |
| 7.1 | 0.8513 | 0.8519 | 0.8525 | 0.8531 | 0.8537 | 0.8543 | 0.8549 | 0.8555 | 0.8561 | 0.8567 |
| 7.2 | 0.8573 | 0.8579 | 0.8585 | 0.8591 | 0.8597 | 0.8603 | 0.8609 | 0.8615 | 0.8621 | 0.8627 |
| 7.3 | 0.8633 | 0.8639 | 0.8645 | 0.8651 | 0.8657 | 0.8663 | 0.8669 | 0.8675 | 0.8681 | 0.8686 |
| 7.4 | 0.8692 | 0.8698 | 0.8704 | 0.8710 | 0.8716 | 0.8722 | 0.8727 | 0.8733 | 0.8739 | 0.8745 |
| 7.5 | 0.8751 | 0.8756 | 0.8762 | 0.8768 | 0.8774 | 0.8779 | 0.8785 | 0.8791 | 0.8797 | 0.8802 |
| 7.6 | 0.8808 | 0.8814 | 0.8820 | 0.8825 | 0.8831 | 0.8837 | 0.8842 | 0.8848 | 0.8854 | 0.8859 |
| 7.7 | 0.8865 | 0.8871 | 0.8876 | 0.8882 | 0.8887 | 0.8893 | 0.8899 | 0.8904 | 0.8910 | 0.8915 |
| 7.8 | 0.8921 | 0.8927 | 0.8932 | 0.8938 | 0.8943 | 0.8949 | 0.8954 | 0.8960 | 0.8965 | 0.8971 |
| 7.9 | 0.8976 | 0.8982 | 0.8987 | 0.8993 | 0.8998 | 0.9004 | 0.9009 | 0.9015 | 0.9020 | 0.9025 |
| 8.0 | 0.9031 | 0.9036 | 0.9042 | 0.9047 | 0.9053 | 0.9058 | 0.9063 | 0.9069 | 0.9074 | 0.9079 |
| 8.1 | 0.9085 | 0.9090 | 0.9096 | 0.9101 | 0.9106 | 0.9112 | 0.9117 | 0.9122 | 0.9128 | 0.9133 |
| 8.2 | 0.9138 | 0.9143 | 0.9149 | 0.9154 | 0.9159 | 0.9165 | 0.9170 | 0.9175 | 0.9180 | 0.9186 |
| 8.3 | 0.9191 | 0.9196 | 0.9201 | 0.9206 | 0.9212 | 0.9217 | 0.9222 | 0.9227 | 0.9232 | 0.9238 |
| 8.4 | 0.9243 | 0.9248 | 0.9253 | 0.9258 | 0.9263 | 0.9269 | 0.9274 | 0.9279 | 0.9284 | 0.9289 |
| 8.5 | 0.9294 | 0.9299 | 0.9304 | 0.9309 | 0.9315 | 0.9320 | 0.9325 | 0.9330 | 0.9335 | 0.9340 |
| 8.6 | 0.9345 | 0.9350 | 0.9355 | 0.9360 | 0.9365 | 0.9370 | 0.9375 | 0.9380 | 0.9385 | 0.9390 |
| 8.7 | 0.9395 | 0.9400 | 0.9405 | 0.9410 | 0.9415 | 0.9420 | 0.9425 | 0.9430 | 0.9435 | 0.9440 |
| 8.8 | 0.9445 | 0.9450 | 0.9455 | 0.9460 | 0.9465 | 0.9469 | 0.9474 | 0.9479 | 0.9484 | 0.9489 |
| 8.9 | 0.9494 | 0.9499 | 0.9504 | 0.9509 | 0.9513 | 0.9518 | 0.9523 | 0.9528 | 0.9533 | 0.9538 |

**Table A.4** (*Continued*)

| n | 0 | 1 | 2 | 3 | 4 | 5 | 6 | 7 | 8 | 9 |
|---|---|---|---|---|---|---|---|---|---|---|
| 9.0 | 0.9542 | 0.9547 | 0.9552 | 0.9557 | 0.9562 | 0.9566 | 0.9571 | 0.9576 | 0.9581 | 0.9586 |
| 9.1 | 0.9590 | 0.9595 | 0.9600 | 0.9605 | 0.9609 | 0.9614 | 0.9619 | 0.9624 | 0.9628 | 0.9633 |
| 9.2 | 0.9638 | 0.9643 | 0.9647 | 0.9652 | 0.9657 | 0.9661 | 0.9666 | 0.9671 | 0.9675 | 0.9680 |
| 9.3 | 0.9685 | 0.9689 | 0.9694 | 0.9699 | 0.9703 | 0.9708 | 0.9713 | 0.9717 | 0.9722 | 0.9727 |
| 9.4 | 0.9731 | 0.9736 | 0.9741 | 0.9745 | 0.9750 | 0.9754 | 0.9759 | 0.9763 | 0.9768 | 0.9773 |
| 9.5 | 0.9777 | 0.9782 | 0.9786 | 0.9791 | 0.9795 | 0.9800 | 0.9805 | 0.9809 | 0.9814 | 0.9818 |
| 9.6 | 0.9823 | 0.9827 | 0.9832 | 0.9836 | 0.9841 | 0.9845 | 0.9850 | 0.9854 | 0.9859 | 0.9863 |
| 9.7 | 0.9868 | 0.9872 | 0.9877 | 0.9881 | 0.9886 | 0.9890 | 0.9894 | 0.9899 | 0.9903 | 0.9908 |
| 9.8 | 0.9912 | 0.9917 | 0.9921 | 0.9926 | 0.9930 | 0.9934 | 0.9939 | 0.9943 | 0.9948 | 0.9952 |
| 9.9 | 0.9956 | 0.9961 | 0.9965 | 0.9969 | 0.9974 | 0.9978 | 0.9983 | 0.9987 | 0.9991 | 0.9996 |

**Table A.5**
Natural logarithms

| $x$ | $\ln x$ | $x$ | $\ln x$ | $x$ | $\ln x$ |
|---|---|---|---|---|---|
| | | 4.5 | 1.5041 | 9.0 | 2.1972 |
| 0.1 | 7.6974 − 10 | 4.6 | 1.5261 | 9.1 | 2.2083 |
| 0.2 | 8.3906 − 10 | 4.7 | 1.5476 | 9.2 | 2.2192 |
| 0.3 | 8.7960 − 10 | 4.8 | 1.5686 | 9.3 | 2.2300 |
| 0.4 | 9.0837 − 10 | 4.9 | 1.5892 | 9.4 | 2.2407 |
| 0.5 | 9.3069 − 10 | 5.0 | 1.6094 | 9.5 | 2.2513 |
| 0.6 | 9.4892 − 10 | 5.1 | 1.6292 | 9.6 | 2.2618 |
| 0.7 | 9.6433 − 10 | 5.2 | 1.6487 | 9.7 | 2.2721 |
| 0.8 | 9.7769 − 10 | 5.3 | 1.6677 | 9.8 | 2.2824 |
| 0.9 | 9.8946 − 10 | 5.4 | 1.6864 | 9.9 | 2.2925 |
| 1.0 | 0.0000 | 5.5 | 1.7047 | 10 | 2.3026 |
| 1.1 | 0.0953 | 5.6 | 1.7228 | 11 | 2.3979 |
| 1.2 | 0.1823 | 5.7 | 1.7405 | 12 | 2.4849 |
| 1.3 | 0.2624 | 5.8 | 1.7579 | 13 | 2.5649 |
| 1.4 | 0.3365 | 5.9 | 1.7750 | 14 | 2.6391 |
| 1.5 | 0.4055 | 6.0 | 1.7918 | 15 | 2.7081 |
| 1.6 | 0.4700 | 6.1 | 1.8083 | 16 | 2.7726 |
| 1.7 | 0.5306 | 6.2 | 1.8245 | 17 | 2.8332 |
| 1.8 | 0.5878 | 6.3 | 1.8405 | 18 | 2.8904 |
| 1.9 | 0.6419 | 6.4 | 1.8563 | 19 | 2.9444 |
| 2.0 | 0.6931 | 6.5 | 1.8718 | 20 | 2.9957 |
| 2.1 | 0.7419 | 6.6 | 1.8871 | | |
| 2.2 | 0.7885 | 6.7 | 1.9021 | 25 | 3.2189 |
| 2.3 | 0.8329 | 6.8 | 1.9169 | 30 | 3.4012 |
| 2.4 | 0.8755 | 6.9 | 1.9315 | 35 | 3.5553 |
| | | | | 40 | 3.6889 |
| 2.5 | 0.9163 | 7.0 | 1.9459 | | |
| 2.6 | 0.9555 | 7.1 | 1.9601 | 45 | 3.8067 |
| 2.7 | 0.9933 | 7.2 | 1.9741 | 50 | 3.9120 |
| 2.8 | 1.0296 | 7.3 | 1.9879 | | |
| 2.9 | 1.0647 | 7.4 | 2.0015 | 55 | 4.0073 |
| | | | | 60 | 4.0943 |
| 3.0 | 1.0986 | 7.5 | 2.0149 | 65 | 4.1744 |
| 3.1 | 1.1314 | 7.6 | 2.0281 | | |
| 3.2 | 1.1632 | 7.7 | 2.0412 | 70 | 4.2485 |
| 3.3 | 1.1939 | 7.8 | 2.0541 | 75 | 4.3175 |
| 3.4 | 1.2238 | 7.9 | 2.0669 | 80 | 4.3820 |
| | | | | 85 | 4.4427 |
| 3.5 | 1.2528 | 8.0 | 2.0794 | 90 | 4.4998 |
| 3.6 | 1.2809 | 8.1 | 2.0919 | | |
| 3.7 | 1.2083 | 8.2 | 2.1041 | 95 | 4.5539 |
| 3.8 | 1.3350 | 8.3 | 2.1163 | 100 | 4.6052 |
| 3.9 | 1.3610 | 8.4 | 2.1281 | | |
| 4.0 | 1.3863 | 8.5 | 2.1401 | | |
| 4.1 | 1.4110 | 8.6 | 2.1518 | | |
| 4.2 | 1.4351 | 8.7 | 2.1633 | | |
| 4.3 | 1.4586 | 8.8 | 2.1748 | | |
| 4.4 | 1.4816 | 8.9 | 2.1861 | | |

**Table A.6**
Powers of $e$: $\exp(x)$ and $\exp(-x)$

| $x$ | $e^x$ | $e^{-x}$ | $x$ | $e^x$ | $e^{-x}$ |
|------|---------|---------|-------|-------------|---------|
| 0.00 | 1.00000 | 1.00000 | 1.60 | 4.95302 | 0.20189 |
| 0.01 | 1.01005 | 0.99004 | 1.70 | 5.47394 | 0.18268 |
| 0.02 | 1.02020 | 0.98019 | 1.80 | 6.04964 | 0.16529 |
| 0.03 | 1.03045 | 0.97044 | 1.90 | 6.68589 | 0.14956 |
| 0.04 | 1.04081 | 0.96078 | 2.00 | 7.38905 | 0.13533 |
| 0.05 | 1.05127 | 0.95122 |      |             |         |
| 0.06 | 1.06183 | 0.94176 | 2.10 | 8.16616 | 0.12245 |
| 0.07 | 1.07250 | 0.93239 | 2.20 | 9.02500 | 0.11080 |
| 0.08 | 1.08328 | 0.92311 | 2.30 | 9.97417 | 0.10025 |
| 0.09 | 1.09417 | 0.91393 | 2.40 | 11.02316 | 0.09071 |
| 0.10 | 1.10517 | 0.90483 | 2.50 | 12.18248 | 0.08208 |
|      |         |         | 2.60 | 13.46372 | 0.07427 |
| 0.11 | 1.11628 | 0.89583 | 2.70 | 14.87971 | 0.06720 |
| 0.12 | 1.12750 | 0.88692 | 2.80 | 16.44463 | 0.06081 |
| 0.13 | 1.13883 | 0.87810 | 2.90 | 18.17412 | 0.05502 |
| 0.14 | 1.15027 | 0.86936 | 3.00 | 20.08551 | 0.04978 |
| 0.15 | 1.16183 | 0.86071 |      |             |         |
| 0.16 | 1.17351 | 0.85214 | 3.50 | 33.11545 | 0.03020 |
| 0.17 | 1.18530 | 0.84366 |      |             |         |
| 0.18 | 1.19722 | 0.83527 | 4.00 | 54.95815 | 0.01832 |
| 0.19 | 1.20925 | 0.82696 | 4.50 | 90.01713 | 0.01111 |
| 0.20 | 1.22140 | 0.81873 | 5.00 | 148.41316 | 0.00674 |
| 0.30 | 1.34985 | 0.74081 | 5.50 | 224.69193 | 0.00409 |
| 0.40 | 1.49182 | 0.67032 |      |             |         |
| 0.50 | 1.64872 | 0.60653 | 6.00 | 403.42879 | 0.00248 |
| 0.60 | 1.82211 | 0.54881 | 6.50 | 665.14163 | 0.00150 |
| 0.70 | 2.01375 | 0.49658 |      |             |         |
| 0.80 | 2.22554 | 0.44932 | 7.00 | 1096.63316 | 0.00091 |
| 0.90 | 2.45960 | 0.40656 | 7.50 | 1808.04241 | 0.00055 |
| 1.00 | 2.71828 | 0.36787 |      |             |         |
|      |         |         | 8.00 | 2980.95799 | 0.00034 |
|      |         |         | 8.50 | 4914.76884 | 0.00020 |
| 1.10 | 3.00416 | 0.33287 |      |             |         |
| 1.20 | 3.32011 | 0.30119 | 9.00 | 8130.08393 | 0.00012 |
| 1.30 | 3.66929 | 0.27253 | 9.50 | 13359.72683 | 0.00007 |
| 1.40 | 4.05519 | 0.24659 |      |             |         |
| 1.50 | 4.48168 | 0.22313 | 10.00 | 22026.46579 | 0.00005 |

**Table A.7**

Squares and square roots

| $n$ | $n^2$ | $\sqrt{n}$ | $\sqrt{10n}$ | $n$ | $n^2$ | $\sqrt{n}$ | $\sqrt{10n}$ |
|---|---|---|---|---|---|---|---|
| 1 | 1 | 1.000 | 3.162 | 41 | 1681 | 6.403 | 20.248 |
| 2 | 4 | 1.414 | 4.472 | 42 | 1764 | 6.481 | 20.494 |
| 3 | 9 | 1.732 | 5.477 | 43 | 1849 | 6.557 | 20.736 |
| 4 | 16 | 2.000 | 6.325 | 44 | 1936 | 6.633 | 20.976 |
| 5 | 25 | 2.236 | 7.071 | 45 | 2025 | 6.708 | 21.213 |
| 6 | 36 | 2.449 | 7.746 | 46 | 2116 | 6.782 | 21.448 |
| 7 | 49 | 2.646 | 8.367 | 47 | 2209 | 6.856 | 21.679 |
| 8 | 64 | 2.828 | 8.944 | 48 | 2304 | 6.928 | 21.909 |
| 9 | 81 | 3.000 | 9.487 | 49 | 2401 | 7.000 | 22.136 |
| 10 | 100 | 3.162 | 10.000 | 50 | 2500 | 7.071 | 22.361 |
| 11 | 121 | 3.317 | 10.488 | 51 | 2601 | 7.141 | 22.583 |
| 12 | 144 | 3.464 | 10.954 | 52 | 2704 | 7.211 | 22.804 |
| 13 | 169 | 3.606 | 11.402 | 53 | 2809 | 7.280 | 23.022 |
| 14 | 196 | 3.742 | 11.832 | 54 | 2916 | 7.348 | 23.238 |
| 15 | 225 | 3.873 | 12.247 | 55 | 3025 | 7.416 | 23.452 |
| 16 | 256 | 4.000 | 12.649 | 56 | 3136 | 7.483 | 23.664 |
| 17 | 289 | 4.123 | 13.038 | 57 | 3249 | 7.550 | 23.875 |
| 18 | 324 | 4.243 | 13.416 | 58 | 3364 | 7.616 | 24.083 |
| 19 | 361 | 4.359 | 13.784 | 59 | 3481 | 7.681 | 24.290 |
| 20 | 400 | 4.472 | 14.142 | 60 | 3600 | 7.746 | 24.495 |
| 21 | 441 | 4.583 | 14.491 | 61 | 3721 | 7.810 | 24.698 |
| 22 | 484 | 4.690 | 14.832 | 62 | 3844 | 7.874 | 24.900 |
| 23 | 529 | 4.796 | 15.166 | 63 | 3969 | 7.937 | 25.100 |
| 24 | 576 | 4.899 | 15.492 | 64 | 4096 | 8.000 | 25.298 |
| 25 | 625 | 5.000 | 15.811 | 65 | 4225 | 8.062 | 25.495 |
| 26 | 676 | 5.099 | 16.125 | 66 | 4356 | 8.124 | 25.690 |
| 27 | 729 | 5.196 | 16.432 | 67 | 4489 | 8.185 | 25.884 |
| 28 | 784 | 5.292 | 16.733 | 68 | 4624 | 8.246 | 26.077 |
| 29 | 841 | 5.385 | 17.029 | 69 | 4761 | 8.307 | 26.268 |
| 30 | 900 | 5.477 | 17.321 | 70 | 4900 | 8.367 | 26.458 |
| 31 | 961 | 5.568 | 17.607 | 71 | 5041 | 8.426 | 26.646 |
| 32 | 1024 | 5.657 | 17.889 | 72 | 5184 | 8.485 | 26.833 |
| 33 | 1089 | 5.745 | 18.166 | 73 | 5329 | 8.544 | 27.019 |
| 34 | 1156 | 5.831 | 18.439 | 74 | 5476 | 8.602 | 27.203 |
| 35 | 1225 | 5.916 | 18.708 | 75 | 5625 | 8.660 | 27.386 |
| 36 | 1296 | 6.000 | 18.974 | 76 | 5776 | 8.718 | 27.568 |
| 37 | 1369 | 6.083 | 19.235 | 77 | 5929 | 8.775 | 27.749 |
| 38 | 1444 | 6.164 | 19.494 | 78 | 6084 | 8.832 | 27.928 |
| 39 | 1521 | 6.245 | 19.748 | 79 | 6241 | 8.888 | 28.107 |
| 40 | 1600 | 6.325 | 20.000 | 80 | 6400 | 8.944 | 28.284 |

**Table A.7** (*Continued*)

| $n$ | $n^2$ | $\sqrt{n}$ | $\sqrt{10n}$ | $n$ | $n^2$ | $\sqrt{n}$ | $\sqrt{10n}$ |
|----|------|-----------|-------------|----|------|-----------|-------------|
| 81 | 6561 | 9.000 | 28.460 | 91 | 8281 | 9.539 | 30.166 |
| 82 | 6724 | 9.055 | 28.636 | 92 | 8464 | 9.592 | 30.332 |
| 83 | 6889 | 9.110 | 28.810 | 93 | 8649 | 9.644 | 30.496 |
| 84 | 7056 | 9.165 | 28.983 | 94 | 8836 | 9.695 | 30.659 |
| 85 | 7225 | 9.220 | 29.155 | 95 | 9025 | 9.747 | 30.822 |
| 86 | 7396 | 9.274 | 29.326 | 96 | 9216 | 9.798 | 30.984 |
| 87 | 7569 | 9.327 | 29.496 | 97 | 9409 | 9.849 | 31.145 |
| 88 | 7744 | 9.381 | 29.665 | 98 | 9604 | 9.899 | 31.305 |
| 89 | 7921 | 9.434 | 29.833 | 99 | 9801 | 9.950 | 31.464 |
| 90 | 8100 | 9.487 | 30.000 | 100 | 10000 | 10.000 | 31.623 |

# Molecular Weights of Selected Drugs and Composition of Solutions

## Appendix B

**Table B.1**
Molecular weights of selected drugs

| Agent | Molecular weight |
|---|---|
| Acetazolamide | 222.25 |
| Acetylcholine chloride | 181.68 |
| Acetyl-B-methylcholine chloride | 195.69 |
| Acetylsalicylic acid | 300.26 |
| Allopurinol | 136.11 |
| Aminophylline | 420.44 |
| Amitriptyline | 277.39 |
| Amobarbital | 226.27 |
| Amphetamine sulfate | 368.49 |
| Amyl nitrite | 133.15 |
| Angiotensin II Amide 5-Valine | 1031.20 |
| Atropine | 289.38 |
| Betamethasone | 392.45 |
| Bethanechal chloride | 196.68 |
| Bishydroxycoumarin | 120.14 |
| Bretylium tosylate | 414.39 |
| Caffeine | 194.19 |
| Calcitonin | 4500 |
| *Cannabis sativa* (Cannabinol) | 310.42 |

*(Continued)*

**Table B.1** (*Continued*)

| Agent | Molecular weight |
|---|---|
| Carbamazepine | 236.26 |
| Carbamylcholine | 182.65 |
| Chloral hydrate | 165.42 |
| Chlordiazepoxide | 299.75 |
| Chlorpheniramine | 274.80 |
| Chlorothiazide | 295.72 |
| Chlorpromazine | 318.88 |
| Chlorthalidone | 338.78 |
| Clomiphene | 405.98 |
| Clonidine | 230.10 |
| Cocaine | 303.35 |
| Codeine sulfate | 696.82 |
| Cromolyn sodium | 468.38 |
| Cyclic 3'5'-AMP | 329.22 |
| Cyclizine hydrochloride | 266.37 |
| Decamethonium bromide | 418.36 |
| Desipramine | 266.37 |
| Dextroamphetamine sulfate | 368.49 |
| Diazepam | 284.76 |
| Diazoxide | 230.70 |
| Digitoxin | 764.92 |
| Digoxin | 780.92 |
| Dihydromorphinone | 287.35 |
| Dimenhydrinate | 469.96 |
| Diphenhydramine hydrochloride | 255.35 |
| Diphenoxylate | 452.57 |
| Diphenylhydantoin | 252.26 |
| Dopamine | 153.18 |
| Edrophonium bromide | 246.15 |
| Ephedrine | 165.23 |
| Epinephrine | 183.20 |
| Ethosuximide | 141.17 |
| Flurazepam | 387.89 |
| Furosemide | 330.77 |
| Gallamine triethiodide | 891.56 |
| Glutethimide | 217.26 |
| Glyceryl trinitrate | 227.09 |
| Guanethidine | 198.31 |
| Heparin | 6000–20,000 |
| Heroin | 405.88 |
| Hexamethonium chloride | 273.29 |
| Histamine | 111.15 |
| Homatropine methylbromide | 370.29 |
| Hydralazine | 160.18 |
| Hydrochlorothiazide | 297.72 |
| Hydrocortisone | 362.47 |
| Hyoscine | 289.36 |
| Imipramine | 280.40 |
| Isoproterenol | 211.24 |
| Isosorbide dinitrate | 236.14 |

**Table B.1** (*Continued*)

| Agent | Molecular weight |
|---|---|
| Ketamine | 237.74 |
| Levodopa | 197.19 |
| Lidocaine | 234.33 |
| Lysergicacid diethylamide | 323.42 |
| Mannitol hexanitrate | 452.17 |
| Mecamylamine | 167.29 |
| Meclizine hydrochloride | 390.96 |
| Meperidine | 247.35 |
| Meprobamate | 218.25 |
| $\alpha$-Methyldopa | 211.21 |
| Morphine sulfate | 668.76 |
| Nalorphine | 311.37 |
| Naloxone | 327.37 |
| Neostigmine methyl sulfate | 334.39 |
| Nicotine | 162.23 |
| Norephinephrine | 169.18 |
| Pancuronium bromide | 732.70 |
| Papaverine | 339.38 |
| Pentazocine | 285.44 |
| Pentobarbital sodium | 248.26 |
| Phencyclidine | 243.38 |
| Phenobarbital | 232.23 |
| Phenoxybenzamine | 303.84 |
| Phentolamine | 281.35 |
| Phenylephrine hydrochloride | 203.67 |
| Physostigmine | 275.34 |
| Pilocarpine hydrochloride | 244.72 |
| Prednisone | 358.44 |
| Procaine hydrochloride | 272.77 |
| Prochlorperazine | 373.94 |
| Progesterone | 314.45 |
| Promethazine hydrochloride | 284.41 |
| Propoxyphene | 339.48 |
| Propranolol | 259.34 |
| Quinidine sulfate | 746.93 |
| Reserpine | 608.70 |
| Scopolamine | 303.35 |
| Serotonin | 176.21 |
| Spironolactone | 416.59 |
| Streptomycin | 581.58 |
| Succinylcholine chloride | 361.30 |
| Testosterone | 288.41 |
| Tetraethylpyrophosphate | 290.20 |
| Theophylline | 180.17 |
| Thiopental sodium | 264.33 |
| Thioridazine hydrochloride | 370.56 |
| Tranylcypromine | 133.19 |
| Tubocurarine chloride | 681.66 |
| Tyramine | 137.18 |
| Warfarin sodium | 308.32 |

**Table B.2**
Composition of solutions

---

*Locke*—(Locke, Zentbl. Physiol., *14*:670, 1932)

| Substance | g/liter |
|-----------|---------|
| NaCl | 9.0 |
| KCl | 0.42 |
| $NaHCO_3$ | 0.15 |
| $CaCl_2$ | 0 24 |
| Glucose | 1.00 |

*Tyrode*—(Tyrode, Arch. Int. Pharmacodyn., *20*:205, 1910)

| Substance | g/liter |
|-----------|---------|
| NaCl | 8.0 |
| KCl | 0.2 |
| $NaHCO_3$ | 1.0 |
| $CaCl_2$ | 0.2 |
| Glucose | 1.0 |
| $MgCl_2$ | 0.1 |
| $NaH_2PO_4$ | 0.05 |

*Krebs–Henseleit*—(Krebs, Hoppe-Seyler's Z. Physiol. Chem., *210*:33, 1932)

| Substance | g/liter |
|-----------|---------|
| NaCl | 6.92 |
| KCl | 0.35 |
| $NaHCO_3$ | 2.1 |
| $CaCl_2$ | 0.28 |
| $MgSO_4,7H_2O$ | 0.29 |
| $KH_2PO_4$ | 0.16 |

*Krebs*—(Krebs, Biochim. Biophys. Acta, *4*:249, 1950)

| Substance | g/liter |
|-----------|---------|
| NaCl | 5.54 |
| KCl | 0.35 |
| $NaHCO_3$ | 2.1 |
| $CaCl_2$ | 0.28 |
| Glucose | 2.1 |
| $MgSO_4.7H_2O$ | 0.29 |
| $KH_2PO_4$ | 0.16 |

*Clark–Ringer*—(In Gaddum, *Pharmacology, 4th ed.* London, Oxford Medical Publications, 1953, p.15)

| Substance | g/liter |
|-----------|---------|
| NaCl | 6.5 |
| KCl | 0.14 |
| $NaHCO_3$ | 0.2 |
| $CaCl_2$ | 0.12 |
| Glucose | 2.0 |
| $NaH_2PO_4$ | 0.01 |

# Calculus

## Appendix C

### Derivatives

The derivative of a function $f(x)$ with respect to the variable $x$ is a function $f'(x)$ defined by

$$f'(x) = \lim_{\Delta x \to 0} \frac{f(x + \Delta x) - f(x)}{x}. \tag{A.1}$$

If this limit is defined at $x = a$, the function $f(x)$ is said to be *differentiable* at $x = a$. The value of the derivative at $x = a$ is denoted $f'(a)$. When $y$ is used to denote the dependent variable for the function $f$, i.e., when $y = f(x)$, we also denote the derivative by "$dy/dx$." Thus, if $y = f(x)$, then $dy/dx = f'(x)$.

*Example 1.* Let $y = f(x) = x^2$. Find $f'(x) = (d/dx)(x^2)$. We have

$$f(x + \Delta x) = (x + \Delta x)^2$$

and

$$f(x + \Delta x) - f(x) = (x + \Delta x)^2 - x^2;$$

187

thus,

$$\frac{f(x + \Delta x) - f(x)}{\Delta x} = \frac{(x + \Delta x)^2 - x^2}{\Delta x}$$

$$= \frac{x^2 + 2x(\Delta x) + (\Delta x)^2 - x^2}{\Delta x}$$

$$= 2x + \Delta x.$$

We next take the limit:

$$f'(x) = \lim_{\Delta x \to 0} (2x + \Delta x)$$

$$= 2x.$$

Therefore, $f'(x) = d(x^2)/dx = 2x$.

*Example 2.* Let $y = f(x) = 1/x$ and find $f'(x) = (d/dx)(1/x)$. We have

$$f(x + \Delta x) = \frac{1}{x + \Delta x}$$

and

$$f(x + \Delta x) - f(x) = \frac{1}{x + \Delta x} - \frac{1}{x}$$

$$= \frac{x - (x + \Delta x)}{x(x + \Delta x)}$$

$$= \frac{-\Delta x}{x(x + \Delta x)}.$$

The quotient is

$$\frac{f(x + \Delta x) - f(x)}{\Delta x} = \frac{-1}{x(x + \Delta x)}$$

and the limit as $\Delta x \to 0$ gives the derivative:

$$f'(x) = \lim_{\Delta x \to 0} \frac{-1}{x(x + \Delta x)}$$

$$= \frac{-1}{x^2}.$$

Therefore, $f'(x) = d(1/x)/dx = -1/x^2$.

The functions in these two examples, $y = x^2$, and $y = 1/x = x^{-1}$, are particular examples of power functions, $y = x^a$, where $a$ is a real number. The following result is proved in calculus:

$$\frac{d}{dx}(x^a) = ax^{a-1}. \tag{A.2}$$

Equation (A.2) is very useful since it permits us to find the derivative without the necessity of using the definition. Hence, $(d/dx)(x^{10}) = 10x^9$, $(d/dx)(x^{-5}) = (-5)x^{-6}$, $(d/dx)(x^\pi) = \pi x^{\pi-1}$, etc.

The following rules further simplify the calculation of the derivative of even more complicated functions:

1. *The derivative of the constant function, $y = f(x) = c$, is zero*; i.e.,

$$\frac{d}{dx}(c) = 0. \tag{A.3}$$

2. *The derivative of a constant times $f(x)$ is the constant times the derivative of $f(x)$. Thus, if $f(x)$ is differentiable and $g(x) = c\,f(x)$ then $g'(x) = c\,f'(x)$ or*

$$\frac{d}{dx}(c\,f(x)) = c\,\frac{df(x)}{dx}. \tag{A.4}$$

3. *If $f(x)$ and $g(x)$ are differentiable functions, then the function $h$, where $h(x) = f(x) + g(x)$, is differentiable and $h'(x) = f'(x) + g'(x)$ or*

$$\frac{d}{dx}[f(x) + g(x)] = \frac{d}{dx}[f(x)] + \frac{d}{dx}[(x)]. \tag{A.5}$$

The use of these rules is illustrated in the following examples.

*Example 3.* Determine the derivatives of the following functions:

1. $$f(x) = 5x^4 + 3x^2 + 7 \qquad 2. \quad f(x) = 8x^{3/2} - \frac{2}{x}$$

*Solution:*

1.
$$\frac{d}{dx}(5x^4 + 3x^2 + 7) = \frac{d}{dx}(5x^4) + \frac{d}{dx}(3x^2) + \frac{d}{dx}(7)$$

$$= 5 \cdot \frac{d}{dx}(x^4) + 3 \cdot \frac{d}{dx}(x^2) + 0$$

$$= 5(4x^3) + 3(2x)$$

$$= 20x^3 + 6x.$$

2.
$$\frac{d}{dx}(8x^{3/2} - 2x^{-1}) = \frac{d}{dx}(8x^{3/2}) + \frac{d}{dx}(-2x^{-1})$$

$$= 8\frac{d}{dx}(x^{3/2}) + (-2)\frac{d}{dx}(x^{-1})$$

$$= 8(\tfrac{3}{2}x^{1/2}) + (-2)\left(-\frac{1}{x^2}\right)$$

$$= 12x^{1/2} + \frac{2}{x^2}.$$

## Products and Quotients

A function such as $y = (x^2 + 1)(x^3 + 5x^2 + x - 10)$ can be differentiated if we first multiply. Thus

$$y = x^5 + 5x^4 + 2x^3 - 5x^2 + x - 10$$

and

$$\frac{dy}{dx} = 5x^4 + 20x^3 + 6x^2 - 10x + 1.$$

If the factors contained more terms, multiplication would be rather laborious. A more efficient method is to use the *product rule*:

*If $u(x)$ and $v(x)$ are differentiable functions, then the function $y = u(x)v(x)$ has the derivative given by*

$$\frac{dy}{dx} = u(x)\frac{dv(x)}{dx} + v(x)\frac{du(x)}{dx}. \tag{A.6}$$

Thus, the product function above can be differentiated as follows:

$$\frac{dy}{dx} = (x^2 + 1)\frac{d}{dx}(x^3 + 5x^2 + x - 10) + (x^3 + 5x^2 + x - 10)\frac{d}{dx}(x^2 + 1)$$

$$= (x^2 + 1)(3x^2 + 10x + 1) + (x^3 + 5x^2 + x - 10)(2x)$$

$$= 5x^4 + 20x^3 + 6x^2 - 10x + 1,$$

the same result as obtained previously.

Equally useful is the method used to determine the derivative of a function which is the ratio of two differentiable functions. The method is given in the *quotient rule*:

*If $u(x)$ and $v(x)$ are differentiable functions, then the function $y = u(x)/v(x)$, where $v(x) \neq 0$ is differentiable. The derivative of $y$ is*

$$\frac{dy}{dx} = \frac{v(x)\dfrac{d}{dx}u(x) - u(x)\dfrac{d}{dx}v(x)}{[v(x)]^2}. \tag{A.7}$$

*Example.* Find the derivative of the function

$$y = \frac{x^2 + 1}{x^3 + 10x^2 + 1}.$$

*Solution*:

$$\frac{dy}{dx} = \frac{(x^3 + 10x^3 + 1)\frac{d}{dx}(x^2 + 1) - (x^2 + 1)\frac{d}{dx}(x^3 + 10x^2 + 1)}{(x^3 + 10x^2 + 1)^2}$$

$$= \frac{(x^3 + 10x^2 + 1)(2x) - (x^2 + 1)(3x^2 + 20x)}{(x^3 + 10x^2 + 1)^2}$$

$$= \frac{-x^4 - 3x^2 - 18x}{(x^3 + 10x^2 + 1)^2}.$$

## Exponential and Logarithmic Functions

The functions which we have thus far considered are polynomials, rational functions (the ratio of polynomials), and power functions such as $x^{1/2}$, $x^{-5}$, etc. Two other functions which are encountered very often in applications are the exponential and logarithmic functions. The derivatives of these are

$$\frac{d}{dx} e^x = e^x \tag{A.8}$$

and

$$\frac{d}{dx}(\log_e x) = \frac{1}{x}. \tag{A.9}$$

For a base other than $e$ we have

$$\frac{d}{dx} a^x = \frac{a^x}{\log_a e} \tag{A.10}$$

and

$$\frac{d}{dx}(\log_a x) = \frac{1}{x}\log_a e. \tag{A.11}$$

## Chain Rule

The rules for derivatives that have been given thus far permit us to differentiate a large class of functions. We still have no practical method, however, for differentiating functions such as $(x^4 + x)^{-2/3}$, $e^{5x}$, or $\log_e(x^2)$. We would have to return to the definition of the derivative and go through the work of evaluating the limit that defines the derivative each time. The practical method is to make a substitution of some kind. For example, if $y = \log(x^2 + 1)$ arises, we define a new variable $u = x^2 + 1$. Then $y = f(u) = \log u$ and $u = x^2 + 1$. Our interest, however, is in $dy/dx$; yet $x$ no longer appears in the expression for $y$. Thus, we can get $dy/du = 1/u$ and $du/dx = 2x$, but how are these related to $dy/dx$? The answer is contained in the *chain rule*:

*If $y = f(u)$ and $u = g(x)$, where $f(u)$ and $g(x)$ are differentiable functions, then $y$ is a composite function of $x$, $y = f[g(x)]$, and the derivative $dy/dx$ is given by*

$$\frac{dy}{dx} = \frac{dy}{du} \cdot \frac{du}{dx}. \tag{A.12}$$

*Example.* We can now find the derivatives of each of the functions previously mentioned:

1.  $y = (x^4 + x)^{-2/3}$
2.  $y = e^{5x}$
3.  $y = \log_e(x^2)$

*Solutions:*

1.  Let $u = x^4 + x$; then $y = u^{-2/3}$ and

$$\frac{dy}{dx} = \frac{dy}{du} \cdot \frac{du}{dx} = -\tfrac{2}{3}u^{-5/3}(4x^3 + 1)$$

$$= -\tfrac{2}{3}(x^4 + x)^{-5/3}(4x^3 + 1).$$

2.  Let $u = 5x$; then $y = e^u$ and

$$\frac{dy}{dx} = \frac{dy}{du} \cdot \frac{du}{dx} = e^u(5) = 5e^u$$

$$= 5e^{5x}.$$

3.  Let $u = x^2$; then $y = \log_e u$ and

$$\frac{dy}{dx} = \frac{dy}{du} \cdot \frac{du}{dx} = \frac{1}{u}(2x) = \frac{1}{x^2}(2x)$$

$$= \frac{2}{x}.$$

The chain rule greatly simplifies the work of differentiating complicated functions. This rule has other applications, however. One important application is to problems involving *related rates*. For example, suppose we are dealing with a situation in which we know the function which relates the intensity of effect $E$ to the drug tissue concentration $x$:

$$E = f(x).$$

Suppose, further, that we know the function which relates the concentration $x$ to time $t$, namely,

$$x = g(t).$$

In such a case the rate of change of effect $dE/dt$ may be determined from the chain rule:

$$\frac{dE}{dt} = \frac{dE}{dx}\frac{dx}{dt}.$$

We conclude this section with a *theoretical* example.

*Example.* It is found that the effect of a vasoconstrictor drug is related to the plasma concentration (mg/ml) according to $E = 100x/(x + 5)$, where $E$ is expressed as a fraction of the maximum constriction. Further, the plasma concentration is decreasing exponentially according to $x = 50e^{-0.05t}$, where $t$ is the time in minutes after injection. What is the rate of change of effect at any time $t$?

*Solution:*

$$E = \frac{100x}{x + 5} \quad \text{and} \quad x = 50e^{-0.05t}$$

$$\frac{dE}{dt} = \frac{dE}{dx}\frac{dx}{dt}.$$

Thus,

$$\frac{dE}{dt} = \left[\frac{(x + 5)(100) - 100x}{(x + 5)^2}\right] 50(-0.05)e^{-0.05t}$$

$$= \left[\frac{500}{(x + 5)^2}\right](-2.5e^{-0.05t})$$

$$= \frac{-1250}{(x + 5)^2} e^{-0.05t}.$$

The result expressed is in terms of $x$ and $t$, and the value at any specified time is calculated easily. For example, for $t = 60$, $x = 50e^{-0.05(60)} = 2.49$, and $dE/dt$ is

$$\frac{-1250}{(2.49 + 5)^2} e^{-0.05(60)} = -1.1.$$

Thus at this instant the effect is *decreasing* (the derivative is negative) at the rate 1.1 % per minute.

## Integration

In Chapter 2 we discussed the antiderivative of a function $f(x)$ and the connection between the antiderivative and the integral of a function over some interval. The antiderivative of $f(x)$, (also called the indefinite integral) of $f(x)$ and denoted by $\int f(x)dx$ is a *function* $F(x)$ whose derivative is $f(x)$. Thus,

$$\int f(x)dx = F(x)$$

or

$$\frac{dF(x)}{dx} = f(x).$$

The *definite integral* $\int_a^b f(x)dx$, ($a$ and $b$ constants) is a *number* given by $F(b) - F(a)$, where $F(x)$ is the indefinite integral or antiderivative of $f(x)$. The function $f(x)$ is called the *integrand*.

The determination of the antiderivative of a function $f(x)$ can be a difficult problem and, sometimes, an impossible problem, in the sense that there may exist no function $F(x)$ whose derivative is $f(x)$. The antiderivatives of a great many functions are listed in extensive tables of integrals which can be consulted when needed. The following short list is sufficient for most of the discussion in this book.

1.    $$\int dx = x + c$$

2.    $$\int af(x)dx = a \int f(x)dx \qquad (a \text{ constant})$$

3.    $$\int [f(x) + g(x)]dx = \int f(x)dx + \int g(x)dx$$

4.    $$\int x^p \, dx = \frac{x^{p+1}}{(p+1)} \qquad (p \neq -1)$$

5.    $$\int x^{-1} \, dx = \log_e x + c$$

6.    $$\int e^{ax} \, dx = \frac{1}{a} e^{ax} + c \qquad (a \neq -1)$$

7.    $$\int \log_e x \, dx = x \log_e x - x + c$$

It is possible to verify any one of these by taking the derivative of the right-hand side and showing that it is equal to the integrand of the left-hand side. For example,

$$\frac{d}{dx}(x \log_e x - x + c) = x \cdot \frac{1}{x} + \log_e x - 1$$

$$= \log_e x.$$

In any particular problem the *constant* $c$ can be evaluated if we know the value of $y$ for a given $x$. For example, if $dy/dx = x^3$ and it is given that $y = 1$ at $x = 0$, we have

$$y = \int x^3 \, dx = \frac{x^4}{4} + c.$$

Substituting $x = 0$ and $y = 1$, we get

$$1 = \frac{0^4}{4} + c$$

or

$$c = 1.$$

Hence, the specific solution is

$$y = \frac{x^4}{4} + 1.$$

In all applications, the constant of integration is determined from some set of conditions such as that in the above example. Our discussion of pharmaco-kinetics (see Chap. 5) provides additional examples.

Integration is always a step in the solution of *differential equations*. In some cases, only a single integration is required (as in the previous example). In other cases, several integrations may be needed. For example, the *linear* differential equation

$$\frac{dy}{dx} + P(x)y = Q(x), \tag{A.13}$$

which occurs in many applications, has the solution

$$y = \frac{\int Q(x)e^{\int P(x)dx} \, dx}{e^{\int P(x)dx}} + \frac{c}{e^{\int P(x)dx}}. \tag{A.14}$$

Hence, a first step is the determination of $\int P(x)dx$, the exponent of $e$. The function $e^{\int P(x)dx}$ (called the *integrating factor*) is a part of the integrand in Equation (A.14). The next integration is $\int Q(x)e^{P(x)dx} \, dx$. The example below illustrates the solution of this kind of differential equation (see also Chap. 5).

*Example.* "Solve"

$$\frac{dy}{dx} + \frac{1}{x}\, y = x^2.$$

*Solution*: The function $P(x) = 1/x$. Hence $\int P(x)dx = \int 1/x\, dx = \log_e x$. The integrating factor is

$$e^{\int P(x)dx} = e^{\log_e x} = x.$$

Thus, from Equation (A.14)

$$y = \frac{\int (x^2)x\, dx}{x} + \frac{c}{x}$$

$$= \frac{\frac{1}{4}x^4}{x} + \frac{c}{x}$$

$$= \tfrac{1}{4}x^3 + cx^{-1}.$$

# Index

# Errata

P. 30, line 2, Equation (2.8) should read (2.7).

P. 66, fifth displayed equation, plus should be minus.

P. 99, Eq. (4.22) should read:

$$\text{S.E.}(x^*) = \left|\frac{s_t}{m}\right| \cdot \left[\frac{1}{n} + \frac{(\bar{y}/m)^2}{\Sigma(x_t - \bar{x})^2}\right]^{1/2}$$

P. 102, S.E.$(x^*)$ should be 0.236. Multiplying 0.236 by the value of $t$ yields 1.01; hence, the $pA_2$ is 7.8 ± 1.01.

P. 189, Eq. (A.5), last term should read $\frac{d}{dx}[g(x)]$.